# Determining the Future of Gerontological Nursing Education: Partnerships between Education and Practice

# Determining the Future of Gerontological Nursing Education: Partnerships between Education and Practice

*Christine Heine, Editor*

National League for Nursing Press · New York
Pub. No. 14-2508

ISBN 0-88737-571-5

This book was set in Aster and Caledonia by Eastern Composition, Inc. The editor and designer was Nancy Jeffries. Northeastern Press was the printer and binder. The cover was designed by Lillian Welsh.

Printed in the United States of America

**Library of Congress Cataloging-in-Publication Data**

Determining the future of gerontological nursing education :
  partnerships between education and practice / Christine Heine,
  editor.
        p.    cm.
    ISBN 0-88737-571-5
    1. Geriatric nursing—Study and teaching.    I. Heine, Christine.
    [DNLM:  1. Education, Nursing—trends—congresses.  2. Geriatric
Nursing—education—congresses.    WY   18 D479]
RC954.D48     1993
610.73'65'071—dc20
DNLM/DLC
for Library of Congress                                    92-49038
                                                                CIP

# Contents

# *Preface*

$\mathbf{B}$elieving that gerontological nursing education was gaining momentum, a wise and forward looking group of gerontological nurse leaders took advantage of this momentum and planned a dynamic national conference on gerontological nursing education held in Norfolk, Virginia in the early part of 1992. These leaders knew that the future of gerontological nursing education could not be determined exclusively by nurse educators. Rather, they planned a conference to promote gerontological nursing partnerships between the education and practice settings.

This book presents the proceedings of the conference by providing an overview of the most recent and current initiatives in gerontological nursing education. The purpose of the book is to disseminate the strategies proposed by the conference participants to continue the momentum of strengthening gerontological nursing education in associate and baccalaureate degree programs, graduate programs, and in staff development and continuing education. Through presentations of gerontological nursing education and practice "partnerships" across the United States and Canada, and through active participation in focus groups, outstanding ideas for teaching gerontological nursing were identified and shared. Summaries of the focus groups and partnership presentations are provided in this book.

The conference planning committee is to be commended for providing the vision for this successful conference. The committee members included:

Sister Rose Theresa Bahr, ASC, PhD, RN, FAAN
Former Professor of Nursing
Catholic University of America and
Former Chairperson of the ANA Council on Gerontological Nursing

Mary Ann Johnson, PhD, RN, C
Assistant Professor of Nursing
University of Utah

Wanda Murray, RN
Regional Director of the National Association of Directors of Nursing in Long-term Care

Karen Walborn, MSN, RN, CS
National Gerontological Nurses Association

Jessie Bryant, RN, MS, GNP
National Conference of Gerontological Nurse Practitioners

Richardean Benjamin, PhD, RN
Assistant Professor of Nursing
Old Dominion University

Ann McCracken, PhD, RN, C
Professor of Nursing
University of Cincinnati Medical Center

Ann Yurick, PhD, RN, C
Associate Professor of Nursing
University of Pittsburgh

Special acknowledgment and thanks is extended to Carmen Flemming, Susan Reynolds, and Shirley Glover of Old Dominion University who were instrumental in implementing the plans to make the conference as successful as it was.

*Christine Heine, MS, RN, C*
*Conference Chairperson*

# Contributors

*Barbara K. Andersen, EdD, MSN*, Associate Professor, University of Tennessee, Chattanooga, Tennessee.

*Mary Ann Anderson, MS, RNC, CNA*, Assistant Professor, Weber State University, Ogden, Utah.

*Phyllis Armistead, BS*, Sociology/Gerontology, Midrise Manager, Norfolk Redevelopment Housing Authority, Norfolk, Virginia.

*Mary Austin, RN*, Director of Nursing, The New Ralston House, Philadelphia, Pennsylvania.

*Sister Rose Therese Bahr, ASC, PhD, RN, FAAN*, Former Professor of Nursing, Catholic University of America, Washington, DC, and Former Chairperson of the ANA Council on Gerontological Nursing.

*Sarah Beaton, PhD, RN*, Assistant Professor, Lehman College, City University of New York, West Bronx, New York.

*Anne Beckingham, PhD, RN*, Professor, School of Nursing, McMaster University, Hamilton, Ontario, Canada.

*Joan Bezon, MSN*, Instructor and Certified Gerontology Nurse Practitioner, University of South Florida, College of Nursing, Tampa, Florida.

*Virginia Brooke, PhD, GNP, RN*, Intercollegiate Center for Nursing Education, Spokane, Washington.

*Jessie Bryant, MSN, GNP-C*, Gero-Nurse Practitioner, Norfolk Redevelopment Housing Authority, Norfolk, Virginia.

*Patricia A. Calico, DNS*, Assistant Professor, College of Nursing and Health, University of Cincinnati, Cincinnati, Ohio.

*Elizabeth Carey, MSN, RN*, Instructor, Mental Health Nursing, Parkland College, Champaign, Illinois.

*Ann Carignan, MSN, RN*, Project Director, Community College–Nursing Home Partnership, Valencia Community College, Orlando, Florida.

*Michael Clark, MSN, RN*, University of Pennsylvania, School of Nursing, Philadelphia, Pennsylvania.

*Brenda L. Cleary, PhD, RN, CS*, Associate Dean, Texas Tech University, School of Nursing, Odessa, Texas.

*Carolyn Cooper, MSNEd, RN*, Chair, Department of Nursing, Parkland College, Champaign, Illinois.

*Janet A. Courtney, MSN, RN*, Professor of Nursing/Gerontology, Faculty Specialist and College Cluster, Representative for the Massachusetts (West) Cluster, Community College–Nursing Home Partnership, Holyoke Community College Department of Nursing, Holyoke, Massachusetts.

*Joan M. Culley, MS, MPH, RN*, Associate Professor of Nursing/Coordinator of the Nursing Career Pathway Program, Holyoke Community College Department of Nursing, Holyoke, Massachusetts.

*Katherine Echevarria, MSN*, Instructor and Certified Gerontology Nurse Practitioner, University of South Florida, College of Nursing, Tampa, Florida.

*Sandie Engberg, MSN, CRNP*, Instructor, Primary Health, University of Pittsburgh, School of Nursing, Pittsburgh, Pennsylvania.

*Janet Feldman, Phd, RN*, Aurora University, Aurora, Illinois.

*Gaye Graves, MEd, BNSc, RN*, Assistant Professor, School of Nursing, Queen's University, Kingston, Ontario, Canada.

*Lorraine Guida, MSN, RN*, Project Agency Faculty and Unit Coordinator, Georgetown Medical Specialty Unit, Washington, DC.

*Mary Ann Haggerty, MSN, RN*, University of Pennsylvania, School of Nursing, Philadelphia, Pennsylvania.

*Gerry Hansen, PhD, RN*, Program Director, Weber State University, Ogden, Utah.

*Lori Hasty, MS, RN, CS*, Chesapeake General Hospital, Chesapeake, Virginia.

*Anne Harrison, PhD, RN*, Nurse Practitioner, Associate Professor, University of Colorado, School of Nursing, Denver, Colorado.

*Christine Heine, MS, RN, C*, Associate Professor of Nursing and Project Director, Model Gerontological Clinical Sites Project, School of Nursing, Old Dominion University, Norfolk, Virginia.

*Beverly E. Holland, RhD, RN, C*, Assistant Professor, University of Louisville, School of Nursing, Louisville, Kentucky.

*Dorothy Jackson, MSN, RN*, Chairperson, Department of Nursing, Odessa College, Odessa, Texas.

*Sandra Karam, MS, RN, CS*, Gerontological Nurse Specialist, Beth Sholom Home of Eastern Virginia, Virginia Beach, Virginia.

*Alfreda Kartha, PhD, RN*, Assistant Professor, Faculty of Nursing, University of Western Ontario, London, Ontario, Canada.

*Keith R. Knapp, MHA*, President, Life Span, Louisville, Kentucky.

*Mary Ann Kolis, MSN, RN*, Instructor, Health and Human Services, Gateway Technical College, Kenosha, Wisconsin.

*Deborah Lautenslager, LPN*, Staff Nurse, The Chambersburg Hospital, Chambersburg, Pennsylvania.

*Joan LeSage, PhD, RN*, Chairperson, Geriatric/Gerontological Nursing Department, Rush-Presbyterian-St. Luke's Medical Center, Chicago, Illinois.

*Marjorie Maddox, EdD, RN, ANP*, Project Curriculum Coordinator and Associate Professor of Nursing, Regis University, Department of Nursing, Denver, Colorado.

*Diane Feeney Mahoney, PhD, GNP, RN, C*, Assistant Professor, Boston College, School of Nursing, Chestnut Hill, Massachusetts.

*Marianne Matzo, MS, RNC*, Gerontology Project Director, Department of Nursing, Saint Anselm College, Manchester, New Hampshire.

*Martha Meis, MSN, RN*, Clinical Nurse Specialist, Forbes Gerontology Center, Pittsburgh, Pennsylvania.

*Linda E. Moody, PhD, FAAN*, Professor, Chair of Gerontology and Director of Research, University of South Florida, College of Nursing, Tampa, Florida.

*Wanda R. Murray, BSN, RN, C*, Director of Nursing, Bon Secours Extended Care Facility, Ellicott City, Maryland.

*Dianne Myers, MS, RN, C*, Gerontology Clinical Nurse Specialist, The Chambersburg Hospital, Chambersburg, Pennsylvania.

*Denise M. Nies, MSN, RN, C*, Adjunct Nursing Instructor and Gero-Nurse Clinician, Old Dominion University, Norfolk, Virginia.

*Lois Obert, RN*, Aurora University, Aurora, Illinois.

*Linda Organist, MSN, CRNP*, Benedum Geriatric Center, Pittsburgh, Pennsylvania.

*Marilyn Pattillo, PhD, RN*, Project Director, The University of Texas at Austin School of Nursing, Austin, Texas.

*Sharon Patton, MSN, RN*, Project Coordinator, The University of Texas at Austin School of Nursing, Austin, Texas.

*Kay T. Roberts, EdD, RN, C*, Associate Professor, University of Louisville, School of Nursing, Louisville, Kentucky.

*Olga Roman, PhD, RN*, Professor, School of Nursing, McMaster University, Hamilton, Ontario, Canada.

*Alice F. Running, PhDC, RN*, Nurse Practitioner, University of Colorado, School of Nursing, Denver, Colorado.

*Annie Samuel, MSN, RN, CS*, Instructor/Supervisor, Coler Memorial Hospital, Roosevelt Island, New York.

*Mary Ann Santucci, PhD, RN*, Aurora University, Aurora, Illinois.

*Susan E. Sherman, MA, RN*, Professor and Head, Department of Nursing, Community College of Philadelphia, Philadelphia, Pennsylvania.

*Kathy D. Shireman, MSN, RN, C*, Director of Nursing, Christian Health Center, Louisville, Kentucky.

*Fay Sims, MS, RN*, School of Nursing, Old Dominion University, Norfolk, Virginia.

*Norma R. Small, PhD, RN, CRNP*, Georgetown University, School of Nursing, Washington, DC.

*Barbara Smith, PhD, RN*, Assistant Professor, University of Pittsburgh, School of Nursing, Pittsburgh, Pennsylvania.

*Carol Soto, MS, RN*, Staff Development Instructor, St. Joseph's Hospital, Flushing, New York.

*Barbara Spier, PhD, RN*, Assistant Professor, University of Pittsburgh, School of Nursing, Pittsburgh, Pennsylvania.

*Elaine Tagliareni, MS, RN, C*, Associate Professor, Department of Nursing, Community College of Philadelphia, Philadelphia, Pennsylvania.

*Linda S. Johnson Trippett, MSN, RNC*, Director of Nursing Services, Ida Culver House Broadview, University of Washington, School of Nursing, Seattle, Washington.

*Verle Waters, MA, RN*, Dean Emerita, Ohlone College, Los Gatos, California.

*Thelma J. Wells, PhD, RN, FAACN, FRCN,* Professor, School of Nursing, University of Rochester, Rochester, New York.

*Marguerite White, BSN, RN, C,* Nursing Administrator, Beth Sholom Home of Eastern Virginia, Virginia Beach, Virginia.

*Claire Wilcox, MSN, RN,* Instructor, Community Health Nursing, Parkland College, Champaign, Illinois.

*Sharon Williams, MS, RN, CCRN,* Staff Nurse, Pulmonary Unit, Montefiore Medical Center, Bronx, New York.

*M. Catherine Wollman,* MSN, RN, C, Gerontological Nurse Specialist and Lecturer, University of Pennsylvania, School of Nursing, Philadelphia, Pennsylvania.

*Heather M. Young, PhD, ARNP, RN,* Director of Community Health, Ida Culver House Broadview, University of Washington, School of Nursing, Seattle, Washington.

*E. Ruth Yurchuck, EdD, RN,* Project Director, Southern Regional Education Board, Atlanta, Georgia.

*Ann Yurick, PhD, RN, C,* Associate Professor, University of Pittsburgh, School of Nursing, Pittsburgh, Pennsylvania.

# *Foreword*

An event of historic proportion occurred in Norfolk, Virginia, January 31–February 1, 1992 when the National Conference on Gerontological Nursing Education, with the theme "Determining the Future of Gerontological Nursing Education: Partnerships Between Education and Practice," was held. One hundred twenty-five enthusiastic nurse educators, nurse practitioners, and nurse administrators came together for the first time and engaged in meaningful and purposeful dialogue regarding issues related to gerontologic nursing education and its future, with excellent outcomes to be furthered in many arenas, both political and professional.

Under the leadership of the conference chairperson, Christine Heine, MS, RN, C, CNAA, a conference planning committee with a national geographic representation, keynote speakers, panels of experts, focus group meetings, and poster and roundtable presentations addressed critical issues which fostered an appreciation of the complexity of the issues inherent in gerontological nursing education with a sense of direction for the future.

The purposes of the conference were:

1. to analyze the current status of gerontological nursing education and determine future research and funding priorities;

2. to determine successful collaboration agreements and strategies for nursing education and practice whereby nursing students can learn about nursing care of the elderly;

3. to feature innovative, collaborative arrangements between nursing education and practice related to gerontological nursing education.

This publication presents the reader with the opportunity to share the insights provided by scholarly papers given at the conference as well as futuristic strategies projected in the Focus Groups during this two-day national conference. These proceedings will have major influences on nurse educators and nursing students, advance practice clinicians and practitioners and, ultimately, older persons whose quality of life will be greatly enhanced through care provided by knowledgeable and skillful nurses who view older adults as partners in health care.

*Sister Rose Therese Bahr, ASC, PhD, RN, FAAN*
*Former Professor of Nursing*
*Catholic University of America and*
*Former Chairperson of the ANA Council*
*on Gerontological Nursing*

# Part I

**Gerontological Nursing:
Partnerships between Education and Practice**

# 1

# Enhancing Gerontological Nursing Knowledge Through Curriculum and Collaboration

## Christine Heine

The challenge for nurse educators, administrators, and clinicians is to ensure that current and future nurses have the skills and knowledge to provide quality care to older adults in a variety of settings. The challenge cannot be met exclusively in the practice setting or in the education setting. *Partnerships* between education and practice are the key to educating future nurses through the presence of gerontological nursing in graduate, baccalaureate, and associate degree programs. Partnerships are also instrumental in enhancing gerontological nursing knowledge and skill of current nurses through staff development and continuing education programs. Identifying, developing, and fostering such partnerships was the focus of the National Conference on Gerontological Nursing held in Norfolk, Virginia, January 31–February 1, 1992. The conference was sponsored by Old Dominion University, School of Nursing. Gerontological nurses in education, administration, and practice from across the United States and Canada were represented in this historical conference to determine the future agenda for gerontological nursing education.

Thelma Wells, PhD, RN, FAAN, FRCN eloquently described the current issues and problems impacting gerontological nursing education and challenged the participants to remove those barriers by developing effective *partnership* plans at this conference.

An important aspect of the conference was to update participants on the significant strides that have been made in gerontological nursing education. This publication includes an overview of these major national efforts. Both the National League for Nursing and the American Nurses Association Council on Gerontological Nursing highlighted their initiatives related to gerontological nursing education. The newly developed gerontological nursing competencies for baccalaureate graduates, which were part of a national consensus conference held at Georgetown University, School of Nursing, were presented. A regional faculty development project in gerontological nursing through the Southern Regional Education Board demonstrated successful outcomes in assisting faculty to integrate gerontological nursing in the curriculum. Both the Robert Wood Johnson Foundation and the W. K. Kellogg Foundation have supported two national gerontological nursing education projects that have had significant impact on how to effectively teach gerontological nursing in graduate, baccalaureate, and associate degree programs. This publication summarizes the Community College–Nursing Home Project funded by the Kellogg Foundation. Mathy Mezey, EdD, FAAN, reported on the Robert Wood Johnson Teaching Nursing Home Project and its impact five years later. The reader is referred to a summary of that project in the March/April 1991 issue of *Geriatric Nursing*.

Perhaps the most exciting aspect of the conference was learning about regional and local partnerships between education and practice that have been implemented throughout the country. Two of these partnerships are described in this volume. Old Dominion University, School of Nursing collaborates with three community agencies so that graduate and undergraduate students, under the mentorship of gerontological nurse specialists/practitioners, can have clinical experiences working with older adults in various settings and in various states of health. The University of Washington, School of Nursing entered into a unique partnership with a retirement community for the purposes of providing nursing services and a clinical setting for students.

The success of the conference stemmed from the interaction among the participants through the sharing of some of the best innovative ideas for teaching gerontological nursing through partnerships between education and practice. A poster and roundtable format were used to facilitate this interaction. A brief description of each of these presentations is included in Part III. This publication is intended to provide the reader with a reference of outstanding gerontological nursing education and practice partnerships.

The conference continued the facilitation of interaction through focus group meetings on four dimensions of gerontological nursing education: graduate, baccalaureate, associate degree, and continuing education/staff development. The groups were asked to identify goals and strategies targeted toward problems and issues in successfullly teaching gerontological nursing. Summaries of the group meetings are provided. The reader is challenged to implement the strategies suggested by the participants of the focus group meetings.

There was excitement and an intent for future action at this conference. The conference will hold its place in the history of gerontological nursing education. Through collaborative efforts of nurse educators, administrators, and clinicians, nurses will be knowledgeable and skillful in caring for older adults in a variety of settings. It is to this end that the proceedings of the conference are published and distributed through the National League for Nursing.

# 2

# Setting the Agenda for
# Gerontological Nursing Education

## Thelma J. Wells

To provide some perspective I shall tell the story of the Hands People. The Hands People lived in the kingdom of Academia, a farming culture. There were three kinds of Hands People: Hands Full, Hands Off, and Hands On. They all lived together in a little village called Ivory Tower.

*The Hands Full group planted a broad mixture of vegetables, grains, and fruits with accompanying Standing Committees, Ad Hoc Committees, and Task Forces to oversee the growth. The Hands Off group planted exotic flowers and interesting gourds with an informal plan of monitoring progress. The Hands On group planted a root crop, heavily vested in types of potatoes, and they were all so interested in growth that each visited the garden every day.*

*The Hands People's garden was growing quite well until the Kingdom of Academia experienced a serious drought. The Hands Full Standing Committees, Ad Hoc Committees, and Task Forces had been so busy meeting to get organized that they didn't notice the drought until most of the other villages in Academia had already developed emergency plans. The Hands Full group decided they had better do a complete review of the problem and withdrew to prepare a report. The Hands Off group picked their few exotic flowers and gourds, and using them as tokens left the village to seek entry elsewhere in Academia. However, the Hands On group had noticed early in the growth cycle that the root crop was not doing well in Academia's soil. So they had initiated an exploration across the borders to Practice Land. Some took all their potatoes with them and replanted in Practice Land. Others moved back and forth across the border, bringing nutrients and water to the root crop in Academia. The resulting potatoes were a marvel, highly valued in Practice Land and admired in all of Academia.*

*When the rains came at last, the Hands Full people were extinct. Rumor has it that they starved to death and lie buried under a vast pile of paper. No one knows what happened to the Hands Off people. A few were thought to have been killed in hostile villages. However, the Hands On people flourished. They enlarged the village of Ivory Tower, renamed it "Research-Based Practice," and helped to advance the cultures of both Academia and Practice Land (Wells, 1986, pp. 11–12).*

Of course, this is a very optimistic tale which emphasizes practice or "Hands On" as the core of nursing. It speaks to divergent views in nursing education and highlights a critical need for a link between education and practice.

To put the Hands People story more in context, consider the Kingdom of Academia. It has many states but probably the largest are Arts and Science, Business/Engineering, and Medical Center. These states exist with some uneasiness amongst themselves. There are those who believe Medical Center is not a legitimate state. Further, Medical Center tends to be a bit too independent. It brings in a lot of dollars but, as some note, it costs a lot too. Medical Center is ruled by the Power People. The Hands People usually organize themselves with the Hands Full Group dominant. Thus, Hands On types are few in number and vulnerable to the dominant group leadership.

Practice Land is in the Kingdom of Health Care with the other major states, Politics and Business. It is ruled by Regulators and Reimbursers, two distinct groups who may or may not agree on the rules.

Life is complex in these two kingdoms. Survival is the bottom line. But this means different things in the two kingdoms. In Academia basic survival is tenure. That is, creating and sustaining a record of scholarly achievement through research. Hands On people in Academia usually have six years to demonstrate this competence which is judged according to common standards for the kingdom. In Practice Land survival basically means saving and/or making money. That is, Hands On People have to compete successfully in the marketplace where time frames are shorter and rules more changeable than in Academia.

The story of the "Hands On" people in Academia and Practice Land is meant to compact a great deal of complexity quickly. It provides a coded, and perhaps protected way, to acknowledge different but equally valid perspectives. The greater the clarity of those perspectives the more likely meaningful partnerships will result.

To provide further perspective this paper will reflect on the "patient people" of focus to gerontological nursing, that is, the aging and aged population. Gerontological nursing "Hands On" people will be discussed noting issues in both Academia and Practice Land. And, lastly, some ideas, thoughts, and hopes for the future will be presented.

It is not news to anyone here that since 1900 the percentage of our population 65 years and older has tripled. Projected growth is from the current 12.5 percent to 21.8 percent by 2030 (AARP, 1990).

The phenomenon of rapidly aging populations is worldwide with an overall 69 percent increase in the 60 and over subset versus a 54 percent total increase during the 1975–2000 year span. The greatest growth in elderly populations will be in less developed regions of the world with Africa (116 percent increase), South Asia (113 percent), and Latin America (111 percent increase), the countries projected to have the greatest gains (Schick, 1986). We should put a minimum of international perspective into education programs. At a leadership level, we should explore practice, education, and research linkages with other countries.

To emphasize another well known demographic pattern, reflect on the 85 plus subset. While now only 1.2 percent of the total population and 10 percent of the 65 and over group, the 85 plus are the most rapidly increasing age group. They are projected to constitute 24 percent of the elderly when aged baby boomers join the old, old* (Schick, 1986). Within the 85 plus subset are centenarians, a group that has increased in size more than ten times since 1950. Whereas

---

*Refers to those over 85 years of age.

in 1986 9 in 10,000 were 100 plus, by 2080 250 in 10,000 are expected to be so (Spencer, Goldstein, Tacuber, 1987). Our knowledge base of the very old is inadequate; and, it is very difficult to anticipate cohort effect, that is, will baby boomers be different than today's old?

Currently the majority of the 65 and over group are active community members and consider themselves to be in good to excellent health. However, there are racial differences in health self-assessment with blacks reporting higher percentages in fair to poor health compared to whites (National Center for Health Statistics, 1990). In general, frailty and poor health increase with age as demonstrated by considering nursing home resident ages. While at any one time only 5 percent of the old are in nursing homes, by age category: 12.5 per 1,000 are 65 to 74; 57.7 per 1,000 are 75 to 84, but 219.4 per 1,000 are 85 and over (Serow, Sly, Wrigley, 1990). It is unclear how or if this will change in the years to come. Rather than trying to predict specific health care needs of future elders, it might be more useful to consider a basic conceptualization to guide education programs.

Elder care needs form an equation. Cumulative normal aging is the starting point. This is the gradual mix of physiological, social, and psychological change within a non-specific time frame and with individual variance. Of course what constitutes normal aging is not always clear, and through research what is known is constantly shifting and growing. Superimposed on normal aging is lifestyle, which should be considered on a very healthy to a very unhealthy continuum. At a minimum this involves diet, exercise, smoking, and stress management. Also additive is chronic illness, that is, disease acquired at earlier life stages and brought into old age. Further, there is always the potential for acute illness; one thinks especially of infectious processes. Remember that presentation of disease in the elderly is often different than in the adult years. Another factor is life crisis. These are developmentally related events that occur in a social context, for example, the death of a significant other. An area often overlooked is environmental interaction, that is, the space, objects, and people which impact on an individual in a mix of positive and negative ways. For example, how much of dependence in dressing is due to poorly designed clothes; how much incontinence or immobility is due to poorly designed chairs which are difficult to move from in response to toilet or other needs.

The sum of all these factors is function: the ability to do all the things a person needs to do, such as eating and toileting, but also the ability to do the things a person wants to do such as smelling the flowers and visiting friends. Function is the pulse beat of gerontological nursing.

There are over two million currently licensed Registered Nurses in the United States, the majority of whom hold two year, Community College Associate Degrees. The 1989 graduation figures display the trend of many years: a decrease in three year diploma school nurses, a continued growth in two year Associate Degree Nurses, and a steady pattern of about one-third of nurses baccalaureate-prepared. It is worthwhile to note that while contemporary BS and diploma students have similar demographic profiles, the Associate Degree student, the largest group, is different. Sixty percent are married, 53 percent have children at home, and the students' median age is 31, in contrast to the BS/diploma students 60 percent of whom are single with a median age of 23. These profiles suggest very different work patterns and career trajectories that will impact on health care delivery (NLN, 1991).

About 6 percent of Registered Nurses hold Master's Degrees, and for the last two years there has been a small decrease in graduates. Less than 1 percent of employed RNs hold a doctorate but there has been a steady increase in graduates over recent years (NLN, 1991). Across the different types of Registered Nurse education programs, there has been a general decrease in faculty FTEs per program from an overall 14.7 in 1980 to 11.7 in 1990. The greatest decrease has occurred in the baccalaureate and higher programs (NLN, 1991). Interestingly, student:teacher ratios are reported as stable across this time span, suggesting that decreased student enrollment might account for the trend. However, informal observation of faculty workload suggests that the real trend may simply be leaner and meaner years.

About one-third of nursing schools offer advanced preparation in gerontological nursing but this varies in depth. There are 28 Master's Degree programs which provide a declared major but across which there is no curriculum standard (Johnson and Connelly, 1990). Put at a simple level, there is no agreed outcomes or curriculum process to achieve an outcome in gerontological nursing as an advanced specialty.

Another 38 programs provide some emphasis in the specialty but this is even more widely divergent than declared major curriculum. There are 15 GNP (Gerontological Nurse Practitioner) certificate programs based in schools in varied relationships to graduate degree offerings (Johnson and Connelly, 1990). It has been 26 years since Virginia Stone developed the first Master's program in gerontological nursing at Duke University. Clearly progress has been made. But it would be foolish not to recognize that advanced preparation in gerontological nursing is somewhat incoherent. Nonetheless, students do select this major, but it is the least popular of the specialties (NLN, 1991). Lots of reasons are given for this disinterest and they are all valid, such as limited and/or negative undergraduate content or lack of positive mentors. But reality is that advanced preparation is in disarray and this must impact on student enrollment.

In Practice Land a continuing problem is the Registered Nurse shortage. While the supply of RNs has grown consistently, it has not kept pace with increasing demand. Vacancy rates are highest in nursing homes but represent more than 10 percent of the work force across all major settings (Hassanein, 1991). With increased complexity in health care technology, management, and decision-making, master's and doctorally prepared nurses are very much needed. Government data predicts a shortfall of over 200,000 in these categories by the year 2000 (NLN, 1991). Since the dominant education pattern for basic nursing is the Associates Degree, with student profiles suggesting that advanced education may be less typical, educators face a major challenge to create innovative leadership programs. Reality is that practice has both a nursing shortage and a leadership crisis.

When we think of nursing shortages we need to distinguish between vacancies, that is, budgeted positions not filled and a failure to budget needed positions. Mohler and Lessard (1991), using the licensed nurse standards for certified nursing homes, found that 34 percent of homes needed more RN positions. Working with nurse experts in geriatrics and long-term care, a minimum licensed nurse staffing structure was developed. This standard determined a need for 43 percent more RN, 23 percent more LPN, and 46 percent more aide positions. There is a massive shortage of nursing staff in nursing homes.

Looking to the year 2000, it is projected that 46 percent of the RN supply will be directed to elder care, that is a 13 percent increase over 1984 (NIA, 1987). Projections reported derive from a criteria-based model developed by an expert nurse panel. In home health care, RN visit workload will be directed to an estimated 2 percent of those aged 65 to 74, 5 percent of those 75 to 84, and 10 percent of the 85 plus group. That translates into over a million home visits for the elderly per year. In nursing homes the projection is for 3.5 direct care nursing hours per resident day with one-third of this provided by RNs. This is a significant increase from the current 10 to 69 minutes per resident day. The expert panel projected an overall need for more than double the anticipated supply of RNs with baccalaureate degrees and three times the anticipated supply of RNs with graduate degrees.

For gerontological nursing in nursing homes, they recommended that 10 percent of direct care RNs be nurse practitioners with an overall need for 19,000 GNPs by the year 2000. As of 1990 there were only a little over one thousand ANA certified GNPs and that included both undergraduate and graduate levels. The panel projected a need for a 1:100 clinical specialist to resident ratio. These numbers call for a significant increase in advanced preparation.

Curtin and Zurlage have summarized an expert consensus conference held in 1990 which framed the context of health care for the decade ahead (Curtin and Zurlage, 1991). Major themes emerged which I have elaborated.

*Payers mean business:* Currently the source of payment is predominantly federal or state funds. However, public out of pocket costs are considerable because private insurers pay a miniscule amount of long-term care costs. Will private long-term care insurance become a payment source in the future? It is too early to know. Currently such insurance is expensive, confusing, and untested. What is clear is that there will be continued pressure to lower costs. Managed care is a growing concept but other trimming, tightening, regrouping concepts will continue to emerge and translate into constantly changing reimbursement procedures. High technology care is likely to be rationed and the elderly are a target group. Home and outpatient services will continue expansion but with increased efficiency measures.

*Decision Making:* Since what is best is debatable in clinical care, decision making is moving to consensus algorithm. This method fits nicely to computers and will most likely link to regulatory and reimbursement mechanism.

*The Public:* While public expectations for health care have risen, confidence in the system will continue to decline. Costs and confusing regulations combined with complex and often conflicting political and social struggles to shape health care will tend to either diffuse or alienate public support.

*Atmosphere:* The health care field will persist in a dynamic, fluctuating state characterized by expanding and shifting frames of reference. Authority and power will move within the organizational structure as external demands redefine critical knowledge. The emphasis will be on measurable outcomes.

*Leadership:* Social repositioning of the physician from captain to team member will continue as the need for collaboration and strengthened alliances grows in the cost-driven decades ahead.

Despite problems, gerontological nursing has some strengths nicely suited to the changing context of health care. Practice advances over the past several decades include certification and development of the gerontological nurse practitioner role. While regulations and documentation create significant workload and lots of headaches, they provide standards and objective confirmation of nursing's contribution. Flux and change yield stress and mental health threats but also provide opportunity for innovation and expansion. Advances in medicine serve to confirm the value of the nurse and hard won multidisciplinary networks provide a new strength to gerontological nursing leadership. Public interest is growing based on positive experience with nursing practice.

Advances in academic gerontological nursing include growth in the literature base extending from textbooks to journal articles; increased nursing research which is increasingly large scale, funded studies; an academic presence on many campuses with valuable multidisciplinary linkages; and significant political expansion as evidenced by membership and leadership in a variety of powerful arenas.

Of course problems abound. In practice ethical issues may be the most troubling in the years ahead. Cost, regulation, technology, and demographic trends will intertwine to challenge our role as patient advocate and comforter. In academia isolated specialty faculty may be the most serious problem, that is, there is probably a critical mass of gerontological nursing faculty needed per school in order to insure survival of the specialty as well as its growth.

A variety of strategies seem useful for the future.

1. While federally funded geriatric leadership awards have been available for some years and nurses are not excluded from all such programs, in reality the awards have been controlled by the Medical Center Power People, i.e., physicians. I think it is critical to acquire federal funding for comparable but separate nursing leadership academic awards.

2. We need nurse-managed model gerontological nursing practice centers. This conference provides insight to emerging patterns.

3. Leadership in gerontological nursing must emerge through the planned collaboration of key groups such as the National Gerontological Nursing Association, the ANA Council on Gerontological Nursing, National Conference of GNPs, NLN Council on Long-Term Care, and the National Association of Directors of Nursing/Long-Term Care. From such collaborative networks will come a powerful group identity. We need to translate this into agreed standards for education and practice.

4. Personal survival is part of reality too. There must be tenured gerontological nurse faculty who hold senior positions at graduate level academic centers. Such individuals form the base for collaborative interaction with other academicians. There must be senior practice leaders in gerontological nursing who, through their success in the marketplace, hold power in the practice arena. While in our past unique individuals have achieved these goals, we must develop and disseminate workable tactics as a common base for potential leaders. We must share rather than hoard our experience by creating pragmatic workshops, mentor systems, and realistic support mechanisms across complex and dispersed settings.

5. Political action comes with the turf, action both within our profession and within the health care system. It is a simple truth that positive change comes from positive politics. We have cadres of gerontological nurses in every major nursing and cross discipline power group. We need to work together and use the power.

The most imperative need in gerontological nursing is for leadership forums. This conference is about partnership amongst leaders. The dictionary's definitions of partner are helpful: A sharer, either of two persons dancing together, players on the same team, a spouse, a reinforcing timber (Webster's, 1977). Choose the image most meaningful to you, but all depict trust, communicating, and bonding toward a common goal.

## REFERENCES

American Association of Retired People. (1990). *A Profile of Older Americans*. Washington, DC: AARP.

Curtin, L., & Zurlage, C. (1991). Cornerstones of Health Care in the Nineties: Forging a Framework of Excellence–A Report on a Landmark Conference. *Nursing Management, 22*(4), 32–46.

Hassanein, S. A. (1991). On the Shortage of Registered Nurses: An Economic Analysis of the RN Market. *Nursing and Health Care, 12*(3), 152–156.

Johnson, M. A., & Connelly, J. R. (1990). *Nursing and Gerontology: Status Report*. Washington, DC: Association for Gerontology in Higher Education.

Mohler, M. M., & Lessard, W. J. (1991). *Nursing Staff in Nursing Homes: Additional Staff Needed and Cost to Meet Requirements and Intent of OBRA 87*. Washington, DC: National Committee to Preserve Social Security and Medicare.

National Center for Health Statistics. (1990). *Health United States, 1989*. DHHS No. 90-1232. Hyattsville, MD: United States Department of Health and Human Services.

National Institute of Aging, National Institute of Health. (1987). *Personnel for health needs of the elderly through the year 2020*. Bethesda, MD: Public Health Service, United States Department of Health and Human Services.

National League for Nursing. *Nursing Data Review 1991*. New York: National League for Nursing Press.

Schick, Frank L. (Ed.). (1986). *Statistical Handbook on Aging Americans*. Phoenix, AZ: Onyx Press.

Serow, W. J., Sly, D. F., & Wrigley, J. M. (1990). *Population Aging in the United States*. New York: Greenwood Press, p. 176.

Spencer, G., Goldstein, A. A., & Taeuber, C. M. (1987). *America's Centenarians*, Data from the 1980 Census. Washington, DC: United States Department of Health and Human Services, National Institute of Health.

*Webster's New Twentieth Century Dictionary*, J. McKechnie (Ed.), NY: Collins and World Publishing, 1977.

Wells, T. J. (1986). Nursing Power: Research-Based Practice in *Translating Commitment to Reality*, pp. 11–12, Feetham S., & Malasanos, L. (Eds.), American Academy of Nursing, Kansas City, MO.

# 3

# Initiatives in Gerontological Nursing Education: The Role of the American Nurses Association's Council on Gerontological Nursing

## Joan LeSage

The Council on Gerontological Nursing of the American Nurses Association (ANA) has been involved in important initiatives affecting education of gerontological nurses. Council activities or ANA programs in which the Council has played a significant role are the following: development of standards of gerontological nursing practice, certification of gerontological nurses, a 1985 curriculum survey, a 1984 practice survey of gerontological nurses, publications, and a meeting with nurses from Belgium. The Council was formed in 1984 following a merger of the ANA Council of Nursing Home Nurses with the ANA Division on Gerontological Nursing Practice. The Council provides an important link between nursing practice and nursing education; it serves as a national network of peers. The ANA first formed a Division on Geriatric Nursing Practice in 1966. The word geriatric in the Division title was changed to gerontological in 1976 in order to emphasize a focus on aging as well as health care. The 1984 purposes defined for the Council were intended to promote the professional development of the gerontological nurse generalists and specialists, to promote the advancement of gerontological nursing as a significant specialty in the field of aging, and to promote high standards of gerontological nursing practice (ANA, 1984).

# STANDARDS OF GERONTOLOGICAL NURSING PRACTICE

In 1967 the Executive Committee of the new Division appointed a committee to formulate the first standards of practice for geriatric nursing. They were completed in 1969 and widely distributed (ANA, 1976a). These standards were revised and published in 1976 with a title change, *Standards of Gerontological Nursing Practice* (ANA, 1976b). *A Statement on the Scope of Gerontological Nursing Practice* was published in 1981 (ANA, 1981). The current *Standards and Scope of Gerontological Nursing Practice* was published in 1988 (ANA, 1988). Council standards are reviewed and revised approximately every five years in conjunction with ANA's Committee on Nursing Practice Standards and Guidelines.

The current eleven practice standards provide important guidelines for education of gerontological nurses since nurses should aim for the model of practice defined by professional standards. These 1988 standards go beyond performance of the nursing process (1976 standards) and prescribe practice as a truly professional endeavor. The standards describe organization of nursing services; require creation and utilization of theory; identify expectations regarding interdisciplinary collaboration; support conduct, utilization, and dissemination of research; require ethical practice; and emphasize responsibility for professional development. Some standards have performance criteria for two levels of nursing practice, generalist and specialist. Behaviors defined for the nurse specialist could be utilized as course objectives for graduate education of gerontological nurses. Examples of process criteria describing nurse specialist practice are the following (ANA, 1988):

- "Performs assessments and records data for individuals who require the advanced assessment skills the specialist is able to provide" (p.7).

- "Serves as a consultant to and educator of the nurse generalists and other members of the nursing service" (p. 7).

- "Establishes programs for families and community groups to cope with aging-oriented and illness-oriented behavior, terminal illness, and the grieving process" (p.12).

The criteria do not differentiate between the clinical nurse specialist and the gerontological nurse practitioner (GNP).

## CERTIFICATION OF GERONTOLOGICAL NURSES

The former Division on Geriatric Nursing Practice supported establishment of the ANA Certification Program in 1973. Certification helps the public and care providers identify practitioners with specialized knowledge; it may be linked to eligibility for third-party reimbursement. Gerontological nurse generalists were certified in 1975 when certification was first offered. The certification process encourages both formal, specialty education, and continuing education programs since renewal requires evidence of continuing education. The ANA now has three options for certification of gerontological nurses, and approximately 9,500 were certified (7,939 generalists) as of January 1992 (ANCC, 1991). Master's preparation is required for clinical specialists and new GNP applicants. With the 1998 testing, generalist certification will require a baccalaureate in nursing degree.

## GERONTOLOGICAL NURSING CURRICULUM

Another Council initiative was a 1985 survey of schools of nursing to determine the current curriculum profile for teaching gerontological nursing content (ANA, 1986a). There was a 79 percent response rate. The 138 nursing master's programs responding identified 56 master's programs with a gerontological nursing major and 43 with a gerontology specialty. When prelicensure programs indicated their curriculum plan for gerontology, it was usually integration of content throughout the program. Single gerontology courses (n = 18) and multiple elective courses (n = 6) were uncommon; all but four of the specialty courses were linked to baccalaureate programs.

When nursing programs at all levels (n = 454) were asked to identify content areas taught, half of the topic areas in the questionnaire were checked by more than 90 percent of all respondents. Some content definitely varied by the type of program reporting. Most content areas showed increasing inclusion in the curriculum as one moves from the associate degree to baccalaureate and on to the master's level. For example, quality assurance content was reported by 60 percent of the associate degree programs, 82 percent BSN, and 95 percent master's.

Data showed that a gerontology-focused doctorate was most often linked with schools offering gerontological nursing specialization at the master's level. Descriptions of faculty qualifications identified that 40 percent of faculty responsible for gerontology education had no educational preparation for this teaching. The majority of schools offered clinical experiences with older adults in institutions; home health and community agencies were not used as frequently. Descriptions of gerontology continuing education noted better availability for clinicians than faculty.

The following are some questions raised by the Council survey (ANA, 1986a): 1) What are the responsibilities of nursing faculty in preparation of nurses for work with the elderly?; 2) Is preparation of clinical nurse specialists and nurse practitioners adequate for their roles and functions?; 3) What are the barriers and facilitators for faculty wishing to obtain preparation in gerontology?; 4) What curriculum content should be taught at different levels of educational programs?; 5) Is it appropriate for gerontological content to be offered via an integrated curriculum plan? By identification of these issues, the Council has encouraged further curriculum investigation by others.

## SURVEY OF GERONTOLOGICAL NURSES' PRACTICE

In 1984 the Council surveyed registered nurses who identified themselves as gerontological nurses from their own 3,500 members (ANA, 1986b). Goals of the survey were: to provide a demographic description of gerontological nurses; to identify satisfaction levels with regard to their current roles, functions, and practice settings; to determine roles, functions, and activities of gerontological nurse generalists and specialists. Responses were received from 2,244 (64 percent) Council members; the majority were nurse managers. Most worked in long-term care settings, especially skilled nursing facilities (36.3 percent).

The survey has had important implications for the profession. Differences were found in the most commonly reported activities by type of educational preparation. Utilization of the nursing process was validated. Data were now available regarding the scope and standards of gerontological nursing practice. Reported differences between nurse generalists and nurse specialists supported development of separate certification examinations as well as provided data for curriculum development. The description of gerontological nurses' actual work also established a focus for continuing education programs.

## OTHER INITIATIVES

Publications of the Division on Gerontological Nursing Practice in the early 1980s reviewed issues related to gerontological nursing education and research (ANA, 1980; ANA, 1981; ANA, 1982). A nursing model for long-term care of older adults was described (ANA, 1982). Recognizing the ongoing need of gerontological nurses for up-to-date practice information, the Council has produced a newsletter (*Oasis* publication ends in 1992), and is planning future publications that will focus on the special needs of gerontological nurses and their patients in a variety of settings. Nursing students will also benefit from these books.

In 1991 the Council presented two educational conferences on utilization of the Minimum Data Set in cooperation with the Health Care Finance Administration. It was attended by both practitioners and educators.

A Council international delegation visit with the Flemish Nurses Association took place in October 1991. In Belgium, Council members observed and discussed nursing practice and geriatric care; and met with faculty of two schools of nursing. The Council Executive Committee hopes to learn from foreign nurses as well as provide information to them that enriches gerontological nursing practice and education in other countries.

## REFERENCES

American Nurses Association. (1976a). Standards of geriatric nursing practice. In I. M. Burnside (Ed.), *Nursing and the aged*, pp. 615–621. New York: McGraw-Hill.

American Nurses Association Division on Gerontological Nursing Practice. (1976b). *Standards of gerontological nursing practice.* Kansas City, MO: ANA.

American Nurses Association Division on Gerontological Nursing Practice. (1980). *Gerontological Nursing: The positive difference in health care for older adults.* Kansas City, MO: ANA.

American Nurses Association Division on Gerontological Nursing Practice. (1981). *A statement on the scope of gerontological nursing practice.* Kansas City, MO: ANA.

American Nurses Association Division on Gerontological Nursing Practice. (1982). *A challenge for change: The role of gerontological nursing.* Kansas City, MO: ANA.

American Nurses Association. (1984). *Council of Nursing Home Nurses Newsletter.* Convention issue. Kansas City, MO: ANA.

American Nurses Association. (1986a). *Gerontological nursing curriculum: Survey analysis and recommendations.* Kansas City, MO: ANA.

American Nurses Association. (1986b). *Gerontological nurses in clinical settings: Survey analysis.* Kansas City, MO: ANA.

American Nurses Association. (1988). *Standards and scope of gerontological nursing practice.* Kansas City, MO: ANA.

American Nurses Credentialing Center. (1991). *American Nurses Credentialing Center Certification Catalog.* Washington, DC: ANCC.

# 4

# *National League for Nursing: Initiatives in Gerontological Nursing Education*

## Verle Waters

The National League for Nursing (NLN) is a coalition of nurses, consumers, educators, researchers, administrators, and other health care professionals. It is an active, multi-level membership organization with policy established by an elected, broadly representative Board of Governors, and implemented by staff and volunteers, in activities generated at the national level and through forty-six constituent leagues. At the national level, there are several standing committees, one of which is the Long Term Care Committee, appointed by and reporting to the Board of Governors. As a past chair and present member of the committee, I am proud to tell you about initiatives in gerontological nursing education in the National League for Nursing.

At all levels the League expresses concern for and commitment to the improvement of education and practice in gerontological nursing. At nearly all the national conventions during the past decade, National League for Nursing members have initiated and endorsed resolutions commissioning policies and activities to expand or intensify attention to gerontological care issues.

Four NLN activities that aim to influence the care, in sickness and in health, that is bestowed or not bestowed on men and women over the age of 65 will be highlighted. The four activities are: establishing educational standards and services to educators; formulating positions on issues of public policy and governmental practice; gen-

erating data to assist educators and planners; and providing publications and other media for educational uses.

## ESTABLISHING EDUCATIONAL STANDARDS AND SERVICES TO EDUCATORS

The educational councils within the NLN, for practical and
diploma nursing, for associate degree nursing education, and for
baccalaureate and higher degree nursing education, each set educational standards for their respective programs through the establishment of criteria for accreditation, and through the formulation
of statements of expected outcomes for the educational program.
The associate degree council undertook revision of the expected outcomes for graduates of AD programs in 1990, and with that revision,
a forthright commitment to the inclusion of gerontological nursing
education was made in these words:

> *"Because the aged comprise an increasing proportion of nurs-
> ing's clients, the nurse with an associate degree is prepared to
> address acute and chronic health care needs of this population."*
> *(NLN, 1990)*

The National League for Nursing takes seriously its historic role
providing forums for nursing educators and practitioners on important and timely topics. A series of nurse educator conferences, held
annually between 1986 and 1990, brought innovation and inspira-
tion to hundreds of nursing teachers, enticing them to join in a curriculum revolution. Because of its importance and because faculty
are asking for assistance now, the League has begun, in 1992, a series of annual conferences on the topic of gerontological nursing education and practice.

A set of conferences with a *think team* format, a function of the
Long Term Care Committee of the National League for Nursing supported by Ross Laboratories, has taken place annually for the past
ten years, contributing to the formation of NLN policy, programming, and publications. These are invitational conferences, addressing long-term care topics according to five year agendas developed
by the long-term care committee. Invited attendees hold leadership
positions within major political and professional constituencies in
elder care. The 1992 conference addressed education as a mechanism of quality in long-term care. This 1992 invitational conference

resulted in publication of the papers presented. The past publications include:

*Strategies in Long Term Care* (NLN, 1988), which combines the papers from three invitational conferences, and *Indices of Quality in Long-Term Care: Research and Practice* (NLN, 1989), an excellent set of papers from the 1989 conference. The 1991 conference papers are in print, and will be available soon.

In the arena of public policy formation, it is important to mention, however briefly, *Nursing's Agenda for Health Care Reform*, which includes as one of its key points the need for long-term care insurance coverage, and promotes the availability of reimbursed care for elderly patients by nurses and a wider (than just the physician) panel of care providers.

## GENERATING DATA TO ASSIST EDUCATORS AND PLANNERS

NLN collects and publishes a highly regarded set of data regarding nursing education. The annual survey of graduate programs yields information about the number of nurses getting master's degrees in the specialty field of gerontological nursing. The newly licensed nurse survey data indicate the number of new graduates who have taken positions in nursing homes.

In addition, through a project funded by the Ford Foundation, NLN is conducting an important study of educational advancement determining the factors associated with success in upgrading long-term care workers from aide or orderly positions to licensed roles, beginning with the LPN level. In two innovative educational mobility programs, and in one traditional LPN program, interviews, questionnaires, and focus groups are being conducted, obtaining quantitative and qualitative data that will be useful to educators who engage in educational outreach to recruit and promote success in long-term care workers who could and should move to a higher level.

Finally, the NLN is undertaking a joint study with the American Health Care Association, the organization of for-profit nursing homes, to collect basic information on the number of RNs and LPNs in nursing homes, their salaries, and relationships between staffing and case mix. The last study of staffing in nursing homes was done in 1985, and that data is dated given the rapid changes in the health care world of today.

## PUBLICATIONS AND OTHER MEDIA

The video, *Time to Care: The Nursing Home Clinical*, and a slender companion book entitled *Teaching Gerontology: The Curriculum Imperative*, report findings of a W. K. Kellogg funded project, the Community College–Nursing Home Partnership. A second new video is *Who Will Care For An Aging America?*, pointing out that the future of nursing is inextricably linked to the graying America, and demonstrating why gerontological nursing holds the key to a new level of visibility and power for nurses.

The National League for Nursing provides, through its programs, its politics, its data searches, and its publications, the assistance that gerontological nurse educators and practitioners need to achieve that power and visibility.

## REFERENCES

National League for Nursing. (1990). *Educational outcomes of associate degree nursing programs: Roles and competencies.* New York: National League for Nursing Press.

National League for Nursing. (1989). *Indices of quality in long-term care: Research and Practice.* New York: National League for Nursing Press.

National League for Nursing. (1988). *Strategies for long-term care.* New York: National League for Nursing Press.

# 5

# National Consensus Conference on Gerontologic Nursing Competencies

## Norma R. Small

The demographic statistics on the aging of the population and the increased use of health care resources by persons over age 65 are well known. As we look to health care reform in the 1990s in the United States, the health care of the older population with its increased incidence of chronic co-morbidities, gives further impetus to nursing educators to prepare nurses that will be able to meet the demands of this new era in health care. Graduates from nursing programs offering a baccalaureate degree are entering a practice arena where the majority of clients across the continuum of care are over age 65 and increasingly over age 85 years. The baccalaureate prepared professional nurse is expected to be educated to provide beginning level of practice nursing—as defined by entry into practice examinations and accrediting bodies, as interpreted in the curriculum by faculty. Unfortunately, nursing education frequently reflects the medical value of curing over caring and societal attitudes toward aging. Hence, nurse educators have not given gerontological nursing concepts the emphasis that the reality of the practice setting demands.

The dearth of gerontologic nursing content in baccalaureate curricula has been documented in several surveys. The general lack of knowledge about and interest in gerontologic nursing of baccalaureate graduates implies that, while objectives say, ". . . across the life span," little or no time is devoted to the health issues of those in the last third of the life span—older persons. The complexity of gerontologic nursing, due to normal biological, psychological, and social changes plus the increased vulnerability to chronic illness with aging, is devalued by society and the health care professions. This is reflected in faculty attitudes, the amount and placement in curricula, its underrepresentation in the NCLEX examination for entry into practice, and the status of employment opportunities after graduation. However, the question of what graduates should be expected to know has been elusive with the lack of consensus on realistic beginning competencies, given the academic constraints and competing content areas.

There have been numerous attempts by individuals and schools of nursing curriculum committees to identify competencies they felt essential for the beginning graduate. These attempts have had minimum success at the local level due to the lack of acceptance by the general faculty which must implement them; and even less success nationally due to lack of effective dissemination and perceived credibility of the competencies developers.

The Georgetown University School of Nursing experienced these obstacles during a three year project entitled, The Gerontologic Nursing Education Continuing Care Project, funded by a Special Projects Grant from the Division of Nursing, Bureau of Health Professionals, U.S. Public Health Service. The purpose of the project was to integrate the continuing care of older persons into the undergraduate curriculum. The first year was devoted toward creating a positive influence on faculty attitudes toward gerontologic nursing. Faculty seminars, which included clinical faculty and clinical agency staff, were used to raise the level of awareness about the health needs of older persons and their own attitudes toward aging; and to increase their knowledge base of gerontologic nursing. Faculty seminars were conducted on specific aging topics, such as womens' issues, and on general interest topics, such as the application of the self-care deficit theory of nursing, continuing care concepts, and curriculum development through competency identification, using older persons as the client focus.

Early in the project, a thorough assessment of terminal objectives, course objectives, course content outlines, clinical objectives, and evaluation was done. It was identified that the terminal and course objectives addressed "the life span," but that instructors implementing the courses actually taught what they knew best or what they had learned in their academic preparation, and took their students into clinical practice sites where they were most comfortable and knowledgeable. Hence, little or no gerontologic nursing content or clinical experience was actually identified. It was determined that specific gerontologic nursing competencies would need to be identified and accepted with specific teaching strategies developed and resources provided before the instructors would integrate gerontologic nursing into their didactic and clinical teaching.

Competency development as a tool to guide curricular decisions was first addressed in faculty seminars conducted by our consultant, Dr. Mary Stull. A competency is described as having sufficient skill, knowledge, or ability to meet one's need, such as a baccalaureate nursing graduate's need to care for older persons.

The project personnel then took on the task of identifying specific gerontologic nursing competencies which should be expected of the graduate of Georgetown University. The project personnel, as did the faculty seminars, included clinical instructors/role models from the continuum of care of older persons: the acute care hospital, a community based agency, a home health agency, a nursing home, and a rehabilitation hospital. With this task accomplished, the task of selling these competencies to a faculty, who already had too much content to teach and too little time to teach, was much more difficult. The need to discuss these competencies in the curriculum committee was not taken seriously. It was decided if the identified competencies had the credibility of national acceptance, they may be taken more seriously. This was the impetus for convening a national consensus conference to identify gerontologic competencies.

A national invitational conference to identify gerontologic nursing competencies for baccalaureate graduates was convened October 8 and 9, 1990, at Georgetown University, Washington, D.C. The purpose of the conference was to gather together recognized gerontologic nursing leaders in practice, education, and administration to discuss and to come to consensus on the minimum nursing knowledge and skills that a graduate of a baccalaureate program should have upon graduation to provide care for older persons, given that the educational programs are required to prepare generalists for a variety of settings.

Since the employers would have a vested interest in having graduates prepared with minimum competencies, corporate sponsorship was explored and met with a very encouraging response. Three multifacility/service long term care corporations provided the core funding with encouraging amounts coming from other corporations. This demonstrated the importance the corporations placed on their need to know and to have input into what are realistic expectations of a new graduate in the area of gerontologic nursing in order to meet our mutual goal—quality health care and services for older persons. The next major indication for a need for national consensus on gerontologic nursing competencies for baccalaureate graduates came from the overwhelming positive response of the invited leaders in gerontologic nursing practice, education, and administration, all of whom took time from already busy travel and speaking schedules to be a part of this consensus conference. It was indeed a *summit* of gerontologic nursing leaders.

The nineteen participants were divided into three groups which had the identical task of identifying realistic essential knowledge, skills, and attributes of beginning new baccalaureate graduates caring for older persons regardless of setting. These groups were facilitated by professional group facilitators. The total group decided to use the nursing process: assessing, planning, implementing, and evaluating, to focus the groups' deliberations. After consensus was obtained on competencies for each component of the nursing process, the groups were brought together to validate the intent of the competencies identified and to come to a total group consensus. An additional category for professional practice competencies was also identified. This provided two days of very intense discussion and refinement given the need for gerontologic nursing in a wide variety of practice settings, the academic constraints of the educational settings, and the regulatory and fiscal parameters.

Following the conference, a transcript of the competencies as identified and recorded was sent to all participants for validation. The comments were then incorporated into the first draft of the competencies done by the project personnel and sent to the participants for validation that the organization and wording did not detract from the intent. In addition, the participants were asked to separate competencies into baccalaureate and master's levels of preparation, as it was evident that limitations had to be placed on the expectations for a beginning baccalaureate graduate.

Dr. Thelma Wells was the keynote speaker for the consensus conference and had set the stage for the work of the conferee as well as the conference organizers by describing the historical attempts at defining gerontologic nursing competencies and the pitfalls to their dissemination, acceptance, and implementation. Using her insights as the road map and her admonishment to not allow this important work to end up on a book shelf where so many other attempts at identifying competencies have ended, work was begun on producing a usable document. The document that has evolved after many drafts is not inclusive of all competencies for baccalaureate graduates which are already identified in most curricula and in, *Essentials of Baccalaureate Education* (AACN, 1986), as applicable "across the life span." Only those competencies which warrant specific emphasis on the care of older persons are included.

During the same period that these baccalaureate competencies were being refined, the associate degree educators were developing the gerontologic nursing competencies for associate degree graduates as part of the Kellogg Foundation Project, Community College–Nursing Home Partnerships. The National League for Nursing (NLN) published both sets of competencies in a monograph for distribution in January 1992. To disseminate the competencies and to assist faculty in developing strategies for implementation, the NLN, along with the Community College–Nursing Home Partnership and Georgetown University, organized and sponsored two dissemination conferences entitled, *Gerontological Nursing: Issues and Opportunities for the 21st Century*. Further strategies to facilitate implementation are being considered, such as a summer institute and the publication of a *how to* monograph.

The very positive response to the identification and dissemination of nationally accepted gerontologic nursing competencies for beginning baccalaureate graduates by gerontologic nursing leaders from practice, education, and administration, and the corporations who employ these graduates, has been rewarding. The time is right to reevaluate baccalaureate nursing curricula to see if the objectives, content, and clinical experiences are really preparing graduates to function in a health care arena that is rapidly changing in recognition of changing demographic and societal needs, and the fiscal constraints of the current high technology, cure-focus health care system.

# 6

## Southern Regional Education Board Teaching Gerontological Nursing Project

E. Ruth Yurchuck

The demographics of aging are well-known. Within the fifteen-state Southern Regional Education Board (SREB) region[1], the aging population is growing at a faster rate than in the United States as a whole. This reality makes it imperative that faculty in regional collegiate nursing education programs increase their knowledge base and clinical skills in gerontological nursing.

For this reason, the Southern Council on Collegiate Education for Nursing (SCCEN) resolved in the fall of 1987 to initiate a regional project on faculty development, *Faculty Preparation for Teaching Gerontological Nursing*. A three-year Department of Health and Human Services, Division of Nursing Special Projects grant (D10NU24299) to support the project was approved and funded in September 1989.

The project model is one familiar to most nursing educators, approaching faculty development through three components: *education*, through workshops and conferences; *implementation*, through workshop participant completion of a project that meets the priority gerontological nursing need of the participant's school or community; and *dissemination*, extending information about project activities through participants and project staff. A description of the project model in operation follows.

---

[1]SREB states include Alabama, Arkansas, Florida, Georgia, Kentucky, Louisiana, Maryland, Mississippi, North Carolina, Oklahoma, South Carolina, Tennessee, Texas, Virginia, and West Virginia.

## PROJECT OBJECTIVES AND ACTIVITIES

The three objectives of the project are to:

1. Provide comprehensive continuing education programs to improve faculty practice in gerontological nursing throughout the Southern region;

2. Promote opportunities for participants to apply educational experiences in their individual schools and communities; and

3. Provide ongoing communication about current trends in gerontological nursing to faculty throughout the region.

To achieve these objectives, a number of diverse educational activities were designed for nursing faculty, including a series of one-week workshops at eight regional sites, participant design and implementation of a gerontological nursing education project, annual regional conferences, and a variety of publications.

Targeted to nursing faculty with little formal preparation in gerontological nursing, one-week workshops were held at eight regional sites (University of Alabama at Birmingham; University of Arkansas for Medical Sciences, Little Rock; University of South Florida, Tampa; Georgia State University, Atlanta; University of Mississippi Medical Center, Jackson; Clemson University, Clemson, South Carolina; University of Texas Health Science Center at Houston; and Virginia Commonwealth University/Medical College of Virginia, Richmond). Each site had a designated coordinator and primary faculty member. The 1990 workshops were pilot-tested at Georgia State University School of Nursing; all eight sites conducted workshops in 1991 and 1992.

Workshops follow a master curriculum plan and, with a maximum attendance of 20 persons per workshop, clinical observation experiences with well and ill elders are included at each site. Use of a modular format allows each site flexibility in implementing the master curriculum. Curriculum modules include attitudes toward aging; the normal aging process; health promotion for older adults; common health problems; health care services; issues in aging; research in aging; and curricular implications for aging content. Teaching of these modules varies at each site, but most are taught by the site coordinator, primary faculty member, or guest lecturers.

Participants attend workshops with the expectation that information gained during this experience will be applied to meeting the priority gerontological nursing need of their specific school or community. They design an *implementation project* during the workshop and are expected to put it into effect within six months of completing the workshop. Faculty from the same school who attend a workshop are encouraged to work together on a project. The majority of participants have designed a curriculum-focused project. Abstracts describing the various implementation projects are in preparation.

*Annual regional conferences*, held each spring, have been highly successful in addressing current gerontological nursing faculty needs in the areas of ethical issues and clinical teaching. The 1992 conference, *Successful Aging—Going Beyond Illness*, highlights the importance of teaching health promotion of older adults.

*Publications*, which are widely disseminated throughout the region, extend news about project activities and provide varied information to nurse educators in periodic newsletters and conference papers. The *Directory of Resource Persons in Gerontological Nursing*, the first of its kind, fills an important need in the region. Based on a 1990 survey of 211 undergraduate nursing education programs in the region, the most recent project publication, *Gerontological Nursing Curriculum Issues: A Regional Profile*, is designed to promote analysis and discussion of content, clinical experiences, and faculty issues in gerontological nursing within undergraduate programs.[2]

## PROJECT OUTCOMES

A summary of some important outcomes of the project follows:

**1. Provide comprehensive continuing education programs to improve faculty practice in gerontological nursing.**

A total of 457 nursing faculty, representing all 15 SREB states, attended workshops in 1990, 1991, and 1992 sessions. The primary teaching responsibilities of most participants have been in undergraduate programs, but faculty from graduate pro-

---

[2]Other project publications include 1990 conference papers (*Ethical Issues within the Gerontological Nursing Curriculum* and *A Framework for Ethical Analysis*) and a 1991 conference paper (*The Demographic Engine—Positioning Nursing's Response to the Future*). An annotated bibliography in gerontological nursing education and compilation of implementation project abstracts are in preparation.

grams have also participated. Increasing gerontological content in their curricula was the specific need most frequently identified.

While the workshops are directed to nursing faculty with little or no knowledge of gerontological nursing, a significant number of participants said they were well-versed in content areas such as the normal aging process, myths of aging, and common health problems of older adults. Participants acknowledged clear deficits in the areas of curricular issues and current research in gerontological nursing, and current issues in aging.

The 1990 workshops were filled and a waiting list was maintained. However, probably because of budget cutbacks prevalent in higher education, every session of the 1991 workshops could have accommodated more participants. Over 85 percent of the participants expressed satisfaction with all sessions in evaluating the workshops. Participants stated the most helpful aspect was the opportunity to interact with other participants and workshop faculty, and noted the enthusiastic, caring attitude of those conducting the workshops. The widely varying knowledge base of participants led some to rate the workshops as too basic, and posed the greatest challenge to workshop faculty.

The ultimate outcome desired for this objective is to improve the nursing care provided to older adults throughout the region. More nursing schools are recognizing the importance of assisting nursing faculty to better prepare students to care for this growing segment of the population. Improvement in the number and quality of health care services provided to older adults cannot occur unless more faculty, who can stimulate student interest in choosing gerontological nursing as a viable area of nursing practice and advanced nursing education, are prepared to teach gerontological nursing.

**2. Promote opportunities for participants to apply educational experiences in their individual schools and communities**.

Of the 53 participants attending a workshop in 1990, 29 persons have completed 21 projects. Over 70 percent of these completed projects are curriculum-based, involving assessment of curricula for gerontological content, development of a separate elective or required course in gerontological nursing, integrating gerontological content throughout a curriculum, or incorporating new clinical experiences with older adults into existing courses. The community-based projects involve establishing clinical services for older adults that are provided by faculty and students of schools represented.

Less than 2 percent of participants attending 1991 workshops have completed their projects, but this number will be increasing over the next few months. Those projects received thus far are curriculum-based.

**3.  Provide ongoing communication about current trends in gerontological nursing to faculty throughout the Southern region.**

The variety of publications produced by the project is one of its most important outcomes. Periodic newsletters, conference presentations, and comprehensive documents such as the profile of gerontological content, clinical experiences, and faculty in undergraduate curricula, are designed to promote interest in and visibility of gerontological nursing in all collegiate nursing education programs throughout the region.

Videotapes highlighting the one-week workshops will be made available to regional schools for faculty development programs in gerontological nursing. Two videotapes focusing on research in gerontological nursing will also be made available to nursing schools throughout the region.

In summary, the *Faculty Preparation for Teaching Gerontological Nursing* project is providing nursing faculty in SREB states with an opportunity to improve their understanding and appreciation of gerontological nursing as a special body of knowledge. The project's aim is to improve the teaching of this important content and to create increased student interest in choosing gerontological nursing as an area of practice and further study.

# 7

# The Community College–Nursing Home Partnership

## Susan E. Sherman

The aging of our nation is no secret. The number of older adults who reach age 65 has increased 24 percent since 1970 and is expected to increase another 44 percent by the year 2040. Dramatic growth experienced in the over-85 population is especially important, because people beyond the age of 85 become markedly more vulnerable to ill health, loneliness, and poverty. In this age group, women outnumber men two-to-one.

Given these population shifts, health care provider education also needs to shift away from the acute care centers, such as hospitals, to centers where knowledge about chronic illness and long-term care are essential. Robert Butler, a prominent geriatric specialist, has said that students entering the health professions today will spend 75 percent of their work lives caring for people over 65. Faced with these factors, it is no longer enough for schools of nursing to emphasize care of the acutely ill hospitalized patient while ignoring the needs of frail older adults in nursing homes. A cadre of well prepared nurses from associate degree, baccalaureate, and higher degree programs must be educated now to provide sensitive and knowledgeable care to these people.

In nursing homes, where the patient population will double within the next thirty years, health care differs significantly from that found in the community and in hospitals. The 16,000-plus nursing homes in the United States provide continuous services to over 1.6 million residents who have functional and cognitive disabilities.

These residents have four or more chronic illnesses as well as more frequent episodes of acute illness than the general population.

For many years, nursing homes have sat at the bottom of the nursing totem pole, afforded a status below that of acute care facilities, and largely ignored by nursing education. Nurses associated with the care of the elderly were seen stereotypically as passive, powerless, and on the periphery of nursing. That sterotype still persists for some in the profession. It is easier to recognize intellectually the aging of the American population and the growing number of clients in nursing homes than it is to change the way that some nurses feel about what is valuable and important in the work of the nursing home nurse.

Consistent with the mission of the community college to respond to local needs, associate degree nursing education—preparer of over 60 percent of all newly licensed registered nurses each year—shoulders the responsibility for preparing graduates who function in the health care world as it is and as it is evolving. It was fitting that, early in 1986, the W. K. Kellogg Foundation agreed to fund a project called the Community College–Nursing Home Partnership, which the originators promised could "show how 778 associate degree nursing programs dispersed widely through urban and rural America could influence present and future care in 16,000 nursing homes in this country."

Five and one-half years have passed since the project was funded, and in the six funded associate degree nursing programs across the United States, faculty and their nursing home "partners" have shown how changes can occur in nursing education and nursing care delivery. Those sites are: Community College of Philadelphia; Valencia Community College, Orlando, Florida; Triton College, River Grove, Illinois; Weber State University, Ogden, Utah; Ohlone College, Fremont, California; and Shoreline Community College, Seattle, Washington.

A wide array of activities have been undertaken at each of the six sites to meet the three major project goals: 1) to develop nursing potential in long-term care settings through education; 2) to influence the redirection of associate degree nursing education to include active preparation for nursing roles in long-term care settings, and 3) to disseminate lessons learned through the establishment of regional resource centers.

Outcomes of the project have been many and varied. These include: production of a videotape *Time to Care: The Nursing Home*

*Clinical*; publication of a handbook, *Teaching Gerontology*; planning of a series of national and regional conferences; networking with many other national groups and faculties interested in gerontology and care of the elderly; completion of a Delphi study which identified essential elements in a successful nursing education/nursing home partnership; completion of a curriculum DACUM (Developing a Curriculum) which identified nursing competencies best taught in the nursing home setting; the description of successful and replicable faculty change and faculty development models; the publication of educational outcomes for Associate Degree Nursing programs and the incorporation of these expected outcomes in the Council of Associate Degree Programs, National League for Nursing, accreditation criteria. To achieve project goals, each demonstration site developed working partnerships with selected local nursing homes to establish teaching centers and to revise the nursing curriculum.

As a result of this project, educators have found that nurses who practice in the nursing home need specialized skills and are presented with special opportunities. Nursing in the nursing home demands knowledge and competence in management, assessment, interpersonal relationships, and rehabilitation.

In this setting, where rehabilitation and maintenance of the resident's quality of life are primary, possibilities abound to provide individualized care and to be a therapeutic provider of care. For students it is an environment where the ethic of caring—not just curing—can truly be experienced. Additionally, the nursing home experience provides a rich environment for focusing on assessment skills, learning about independent practice, management, and the value of health maintenance.

In the process of bringing together the unique cultures of nursing faculty and nursing home staff, creative strategies and alliances which enhance a caring, educative environment have evolved. Outcomes of the collective experiences of faculty, students, and nursing staff support the development of a new community of nurses concerned with health care needs of the elderly. Because of efforts like the Community College–Nursing Home Partnership, the nursing home is now being viewed as an environment where nurses can truly promote the rehabilitation potential of older adults and where students, nursing home staff, and faculty can collaborate within a nursing model which applauds an individualized, holistic approach. This is a model where caring, the essence of nursing, can be experienced and known by nursing students.

Project faculty involved with dissemination efforts to share lessons learned with nursing faculty nationally, are committed to the development of a core of nurses who are vitally concerned with the health care needs of the frail older adult, regardless of their cure potential. This commitment is shared by both nursing faculty and nursing home staff and will form the basis for tomorrow's nurse— one who chooses to make a difference in the lives of older adults in the nursing home.

# 8

## Model Gerontological
## Clinical Sites Project

### Christine Heine

In the summer of 1989, Old Dominion University School of Nursing received funding from the Division of Nursing, U.S. Health and Human Services, to develop and implement three model gerontological clinical sites for the undergraduate and graduate programs. The impetus for submitting this grant proposal was related to the limited clinical experiences available to students with older adults in various states of health and in a variety of settings. Prior to this grant, students had a gerontological clinical experience during their senior year with residents in a nursing home. Graduate students did not have any formal clinical experiences with the older adult. Another dilemma was that there were no gerontological nurses in advanced practice providing services to older adults in the community, consequently, graduate students, in particular, had few options for gerontological clinical experiences.

The Model Gerontological Clinical Sites project has enabled the school of nursing to ensure that all undergraduate students have clinical experiences in working with the well, acutely-ill, and chronically-ill older adult in settings where there is a gerontological nurse specialist or practitioner (GNS/P). The GNS/P is an employee of the clinical agency. In addition to providing advanced nursing services to older adults in that agency, the GNS/P works with and serves as a clinical preceptor for students from the school of nursing.

The model site focusing on the well older adult are four mid-rise apartments owned and operated by Norfolk Redevelopment and

Housing Authority. Each of the four HUD subsidized apartments have approximately 100 apartments and the average age of the occupants is 77 years. Approximately 20 percent are over the age of 85. There are about two-thirds more females than males in the apartments and the great majority are Afro-American. At least half of the residents are widowed with another fourth single or divorced.

The GNP providing services in the four mid-rise apartments, uses a case management approach with many of the residents. The residents' physically related problems are often compounded by financial, social, and psychological issues. In addition to coordinating resources in the community so that residents' needs can be met, the GNP provides health counseling and teaching, complete physical examinations, assessment and/or treatment of minor acute care problems, and management of chronic conditions. A wealth of clinical experiences for nursing students is available, now that nursing services have been established in these mid-rise apartments.

All nurse practitioner students spend half of a semester with the GNP. The apartments have been used for sophomore level students to focus on wellness for the individual client, practice beginning assessment skills, develop therapeutic relationships, and enhance interpersonal skills. Registered nurse students learn about chronic illnesses through clinical experiences in this setting. For example, the students developed an assessment guideline for hypertension, used the guideline with residents and then developed a group education program based on the findings from their assessments.

The model site focusing on the acutely-ill older adult is Chesapeake General Hospital, a 260-bed community hospital of which 50 percent of the adult inpatient population is over 65 years old. The GNS in this setting influences nursing care of hospitalized older adults through regular rounds on targeted units, staff development programs, development and implementation of protocols for problems specific to hospitalized older adults, and individual consultation with nurses, family members, and patients. Graduate and undergraduate nursing students have the opportunity to work with the GNS in learning about the unique needs of acutely-ill older adults. Junior level students who have an adult nursing rotation in the hospital have at least a one-day experience with the GNS. The GNS serves as a consultant to the faculty member and the students. For example, the GNS assists the students with their assessment of the older adult, planning for discharge, and identifying problems for which the older adult is at-risk.

Beth Sholom of Eastern Virginia, which is the third model site focuses on the chronically-ill, institutionalized older adult. This non-profit home has 120 beds. The majority of the residents are judged to have complex, multiple nursing needs requiring assessment, planning, implementation, and evaluation by professional nurses. The expertise of the GNS employed in this long-term care facility, is used primarily to ensure that the special nursing needs of the residents are identified and appropriate care is planned and provided. The GNS, as the liaison between the medical and nursing staff, follows up on residents that require medical evaluation and treatment and does regular rounds for targeted problems experienced by institutionalized older adults.

The GNS works as a clinical faculty member with senior level students as well as a preceptor to undergraduate and graduate nursing students. The clinical experience for the senior level students has been well developed. This is the eighth year that senior level students have a gerontological clinical rotation at the facility. Through the years, a variety of student experiences have been developed. For example, students always are assigned to at least one resident that presents with multiple, complex nursing care needs. The students are expected to be able to develop a plan of care based on a comprehensive assessment of the resident. Recently, students have been assigned to residents that have some of the more common problems found with nursing home residents: incontinence, dementia, immobility, nutritional problems, powerlessness. Students are expected to do comprehensive assessment related to the targeted problem. In addition, students have used the Standards of Gerontological Nursing Practice to conduct a quality assurance review, participated in the team leading experience, worked with the nursing administration staff, and participated in interdisciplinary care planning. In the last two years, the clinical experience has included a collaborative project between students, staff, and faculty addressing a mutually identified clinical problem. Students and staff developed and implemented a Bowel Management Program for residents who experienced bowel incontinence and constipation. Students and staff are working on a program to reduce and/or eliminate urine incontinence by applying some of the strategies developed through recent nursing research.

Evaluation of this project has three dimensions. The primary focus is on students. The outcome criteria is that students have knowledge and skills in caring for older adults in various states of health and in a variety of settings. Another focus is on outcomes in the setting, both from the clients' perspective and the staff's perspective. While the latter has been the most difficult to collect, there is strong anecdotal evidence that the collaboration between the school of nursing and the three model clinical sites has positively affected the clients' well being and the nursing staff's knowledge and attitudes about older adults.

The most exciting aspect of this project is that an educational institution and three practice settings are collaborating to successfully provide nursing students with experiences to learn about caring for older adults. While collaboration is not easy and requires constant attention from everyone involved in this project, the benefits to faculty, staff, and students is invaluable.

# 9

## Partners in Care
## in a Retirement Community

Linda S. Johnson Trippett
Heather M. Young

## PARTNERSHIP IN THE DEVELOPMENT
## OF A COMMUNITY

Ida Culver House Broadview is a retirement community that offers three levels of care, independent living, assisted living, and skilled nursing. It is located in north Seattle and is a collaborative project between an affinity group (the Seattle Education Auxiliary), a private developer (Broadview Development Associates, II), and the University of Washington School of Nursing.

The Seattle Education Auxiliary had a vision for retirement housing for their constituents, therefore the project was developed with retired teachers and their relatives in mind, although the community is open to the general public. The developers brought a vision of hospitality and gracious living to the project and the School of Nursing brought a vision of innovative health care design. The architectural-design features and the programs developed reflect the collective vision of this unique partnership.

Ida Culver House Broadview was created to promote the health and well-being of individuals and enhance their functioning within a residential community. The intent is to provide a warm and hospitable environment for residents that is supported by health care programming and fosters staff growth and development. With the problems of recruitment and retention, there are many opportunities for innovation and enrichment that serve both residents and staff. A shared governance model for nursing management is used in which staff participate in decisions according to their scope of practice. The central focus is enhancing quality of life through care that blends the best of the sciences and humanities. Open communication, teamwork, mutual respect, recognition and continuous improvement of each person's capabilities ensure a climate of caring and a balance of rights and responsibilities.

Ida Culver House Broadview is a rental project that offers the flexibility of matching the needs and abilities of the residents with the resources of the environment (physical, social and functional). Residents may enter the community at any level of care and are free to move within the campus according to their changing needs and abilities. Independent living includes 207 apartments and 8 cottages, the Assisted Living program includes 30 apartments, and the Nursing Care Center includes 74 skilled nursing beds.

Several architectural and environmental features enhance the quality of lives of the residents. On the lovely landscaped grounds, raised beds are available for residents to work with our horticultural therapist. The public areas on the campus reflect the developer's attention to creating a warm and comfortable residential setting through design, furnishings, and decor. The dining room has a wonderful view of Puget Sound, green trees and water, which for many Seattle retirees is both comforting and reinforcing. The library was developed by the residents, who with their interest in education had many ideas about how to catalogue and organize the books. Access to the five buildings is through glassed skybridges necessitated by the inclement Seattle weather, facilitating movement between buildings. These skybridges also symbolize bridging the gaps between different levels of care in our effort to create a caring community. Adjacent to the unit for residents with cognitive impairment, there is an enclosed garden area with a circular walkway for outside exposure. These design features maximize resident functioning throughout the campus and promote interactions and social involvement among residents who share common interest and abilities.

## PARTNERSHIP IN CARE DELIVERY

The overriding concept for the project is *Partners in Care*. Partnerships exist in many ways and at multiple levels from the care delivery level, through program design and through interorganizational relationships. Partners in Care is defined as: "sharing collaborative practice goals and using self-governance strategies to design and deliver high quality care."

The model for partners in care is resident-focused with the primary nurses leaders working together to plan individualized care. The team also includes social services, rehabilitation services, the unit manager (who handles non-clinical activities), the family, nutritional services, and medical services. The partners-in-care team is supported by advanced practice nursing consultation from a Gerontological Nurse Practitioner, clinical specialists in long-term care planning and gerontology, and our extensive faculty consultation.

The Director of Nursing Services and the Director of Community Health collaborate campus-wide in program development. Both have faculty appointments in the School of Nursing and interface with the Steering Committee at the School of Nursing for program design. The Director of Community Health's main focus is out of the Wellness Clinic, providing outpatient services and coordinating community health programs. In the Wellness Clinic, pre-admission screening, health promotion and education, case management, and direct care which includes routine foot care, and subcontracted services (podiatry, dentistry, optometry) is offered. The Director of Nursing Services' main focus is the Nursing Care Center. The Nursing Care Center (skilled nursing facility) has two floors which are programmatically specialized with different philosophies and approaches, one for residents with cognitive impairment and the other for residents who need rehabilitative or restorative care.

## PARTNERSHIPS WITH THE SCHOOL OF NURSING

The benefits of a reciprocal relationship between the University of Washington School of Nursing and the retirement community are many, and include practice, educational, and research possibilities.

*Benefits for Practice:*  Within the retirement community there are numerous opportunities for student and faculty practice. The School of Nursing recently obtained a Training Grant for care of older adults which includes programs for Gerontological Nurse Practitioners. The Wellness Clinic offers the opportunity for the development of reimbursable outpatient practice for faculty. Faculty contribute community service in the form of lectures to staff and residents, leading small groups for residents (e.g., situational adjustment for newcomers), and a pet visitation program. Faculty involvement enhances visibility and participation in the health care community.

*Benefits for Education:* The retirement community has great potential for development of a clinical site, in that the University of Washington School of Nursing has a commitment to developing their gerontological programs with the establishment for the Center for Care of Older Adults, a multidisciplinary group who will be seeking research support and training grants. Clinical learning opportunities are under development to include other health sciences departments such as dentistry, pharmacy, social work, rehabilitation services, and medicine.

The benefits of the partnership with a School of Nursing to the facility staff are significant through courses on site, facilitating staff access to courses, providing career counseling, and sharing educational programs. Faculty provide consultation for specific facets of care (e.g., diabetic care), mentorship, and involvement in our health care committees, specifically research and ethics. Graduate students, through special projects, further enrich our environment.

*Benefits for Research:* Several joint grant proposals have been generated with members of Ida Culver House Broadview staff and University of Washington faculty, particularly intervention studies in which staff may participate in data collection and implementation of study protocols. Active grants provide the opportunity for sharing staff. This opportunity for clinicians to participate in research is unusual and exciting and can be a positive recruitment tool.

The partnership enhances dissemination of research findings. Faculty can share recent findings with staff and assist them in interpreting and implementing results of research. Research collaboration is fostered by the generation of questions by clinicians who can identify clinical priorities for urgent study. The site is familiar to faculty and provides a controlled environment for a study site. Faculty may more readily apply their proposals to this site because of their understanding and involvement. Faculty access is facilitated by the relationship.

*Potential Benefits of the Partnership:* The collaboration of direct care providers with an academic program can promote state of the art care for older adults. While no one wants to move into a nursing home, the intent is to enhance grace and dignity for aging people, by supporting choices and questioning past ways of providing service so that resident-centered, cost-effective programs can be tested and implemented. The reciprocal relationship between practice and academia offers innovative solutions to challenges faced in providing care during difficult economic times with the increasing demands seen in our society for long-term care options. As our population ages and we see an increase in morbidity and functional dependence, our long-term care system must address the multiple care needs in creative ways. This allows pooling of intellect, monies, and energy in a synergistic fashion that is beneficial to all parties.

The partnership increases recognition and valuing of gerontology as a focus for nursing practice. Long-term care is not a glamorous choice for new graduates who are seeking the challenge and excitement of highly technical environments. This may be related to societal values in which older people are less appreciated. Through our collaboration and exposure of students to a positive clinical environment, the hope is to improve recruitment into gerontological nursing. Academic affiliation is an attraction for staff who want to pursue professional development and has enhanced the ability to recruit quality staff. While the benefits of the partnership are many, the ultimate recipients of the benefits are and should be the facility's residents.

# Part II

## Summaries of Focus Groups

# 10

# Issues and Recommendations for Graduate Education in Gerontological Nursing

## Diane Mahoney

Four thematic topics were identified during the focus group discussion on graduate education in gerontological nursing: 1) role evolution of the gerontological nurse in advanced practice; 2) marketplace demand for graduates; 3) regulations affecting education and practice; and 4) the future direction of gerontological nursing. Each of these areas will be highlighted, however, the focus group summary paper cannot convey the excitement generated by the participants who energetically contributed, analyzed, and debated the issues.

## ROLE EVOLUTION OF GERONTOLOGICAL NURSES IN ADVANCED PRACTICE

As universities experience increasing financial constraints, nurse educators confront pressures to reduce or eliminate costly programs. Faculty reported their schools can no longer afford to offer separate programs for both clinical nurse specialists (CNS) and nurse practitioners (NPs). These dual programs experienced more difficulty recruiting students into CNS programs than NP programs and even greater difficulty for gerontological concentrations in comparison to other specialties. Should the CNS be merged into the NP role? Faculty noted that some students do not want to practice in the diagnostic or treatment role commonly associated with NP practice. Other students, however, see the NP role as an advantage offering greater job mobility, status, income, and autonomy, especially in states with NP reimbursement and prescription writing privileges. Yet, in practice, both CNS and NPs adapt to the needs in the employment setting and frequently demonstrate similar areas of clinical expertise in gerontological nursing practice.

The growing recognition of overlap between the two roles suggests that efficiencies may be gained by developing common core courses. One proposal suggested having a three semester core program for both CNS and NPs. NPs would attend an additional semester for an intensive clinical practicum. If desired, a CNS could return at a later date and complete the fourth semester to become a Nurse Practitioner. One university prepares clinical specialists in primary health care of older adults. This title gives graduates the flexibility to choose either role. Two programs reported that they prepare neither CNS nor NP, but offer a functional role in administration or education with a clinical concentration in gerontological nursing.

Although it appeared that the program models were quite distinct, the concept of advanced practice in gerontological nursing was a common thread. Are the differences among programs more imagined than real? Perhaps the critical question we should be asking is: What are the core competencies expected from gerontological nurses in the advanced practice role? Participants agreed that we must clarify our educational product so applicants will choose programs that meet their needs, employers will know what to expect from the advanced practice role, and faculty can improve on program evaluation. The group's recommendation and action strategy was that competencies for gerontological nurses in advanced practice be developed. The focus group members volunteered to serve as an expert panel and participate in a Delphi survey to establish consensus on the competencies.

## MARKETPLACE DEMAND FOR GRADUATES

Participants reported that employers are looking for flexible workers with multiple skills. Master's level clinicians are responsible for supervising others, establishing or contending with budgetary limitations, and providing educational programs for staff and consumers. No longer can clinicians in advanced practice exclusively focus on clinical issues. Rather, they need basic skills in administration and education in order to financially survive and respond to the needs of the workplace.

The group's second recommendation was for graduate programs to offer an overview course in which clinicians can learn basic administration and educational skills, but not at the depth of those who major in these subjects. One course increases the probability that the subject will be adopted into the curriculum (even as an elective) without increasing the longevity of the program.

Another emerging health care trend is the use of NPs in acute care settings. States are starting to limit the number of hours interns and residents can work, and hospitals are employing NPs and Physicians' Assistants for medical coverage. Participants from these areas raised concerns that nurse administrators are not positioning themselves to advocate for and maintain control of nurses in advanced practice. Due to the need for medical coverage and its reimbursable nature, physicians may usurp advanced nursing practice. A task force from the focus group will conduct a survey to identify nursing administration organizations and determine if gerontological nurses in advanced practice are part of their membership. The findings will be reported in an article that will encourage a dialogue between gerontological nurses and nurse administrators about issues affecting clinical practice.

## REGULATIONS THAT AFFECT PRACTICE AND EDUCATION

At the governmental level, the availability of federal funding for graduate education, as well as federal and state policies that allow third party reimbursement and prescription writing for nurses in advanced practice, are crucial. These initiatives promote program development and student recruitment. The group recommended that nursing organizations and programs aggressively and collectively support state and federal policies that favor nurses in advanced practice.

Within academe, the State Board of Registration in Nursing, external accreditation criteria, and the culture of the university program all influence (and sometimes stymie) curriculum reform. Strikingly, participants agreed that the traditional graduate curriculum model is outdated. Part of the difficulty in including gerontology in the nursing curriculum stems from the fact that the medical specialties model from the sixties is still used. There is a need to envision nurses' roles for the nineties and beyond. An emphasis on client function may be worth considering. For example, nurses promote the development, maintenance, and restoration of functional ability across the lifespan. Such an approach would naturally integrate gerontology as a core component and include the often neglected health promotion and disease prevention aspects of gerontological nursing.

In addition, the point was made that we need to value the Master's level nurse as the expert nurse clinician who translates research findings into clinical practice. The Master's level nurse alerts doctoral level nurse researchers about what does and does not work in practice. Master's level research needs to have an applied clinical focus which emphasizes precise measures and tools relevant to improving clinical practice. Practitioners requested that nursing research courses encourage analyses of the cost effectiveness and efficacy of nursing care practices. Also, concerns were raised about the increasing difficulty of interpreting nursing research publications. The group recommended that the American Association of Colleges of Nursing (AACN) be informed of the curriculum discussion and request that they sponsor a consensus forum on revamping graduate nursing education by 1994.

## A VISION FOR THE FUTURE

Gerontological nursing will be integrated in all levels of nursing education. Gerontological nurses in advanced practice will outreach to consumers when they are well and help them to age successfully by offering health promotion and disease prevention programs. In times of illness, these nurse specialists will assess and manage geriatric primary care problems and maintain responsibility for case management when referrals to other clinicians are made. They will remain advocates for the client and their caregiving network, helping them to adapt to life's challenges and endings. As the health care system changes, nurses in advanced practice will acquire new responsibilities for care management and quality improvement. Partnerships between nurses in education and clinical practice will advance the study, research, and delivery of nursing care. Let us now move forward to reach this vision!

# 11

## Issues and Recommendations for Baccalaureate Education in Gerontological Nursing

### M. Catherine Wollman

**P**articipants involved in the focus group discussion on baccalaureate education in gerontological nursing reflected geographic diversity. Significant diversity of gerontological curricula issues emerged from this group, as well. A few nursing schools reflected strong gerontologic presence with several identified faculty having expertise in gerontology and significant gerontological content present in the undergraduate curriculum. Other faculty identified themselves as a singular presence in their schools of nursing without adequate support to meet theoretical or clinical gerontological objectives for undergraduate students. The group expressed additional concern for baccalaureate programs where there were no identified gerontological faculty members.

## PRIMARY TASK OF FOCUS GROUP

The focus group's primary mission reflected the ongoing and significant evidence that there is a distinct body of knowledge related to the aged person that is essential for the preparation of practitioners of nursing in order to provide safe, comprehensive care to the older adult. Recent data suggests that graduates of nursing programs today will spend 75 percent of their working lives treating people over 65 years of age. The focus group agreed that there is an immediate imperative to have minimal standards within schools of nursing that reflect the changing demographic and health care scene.

## OBJECTIVES TO ACHIEVE MINIMAL STANDARDS OF GERONTOLOGICAL EDUCATION

1. *Obtain the support of the National League for Nursing, the accrediting body of schools of nursing.* The group strongly believed that it is now necessary to change the criterion for theoretical and clinical learning activities (Criterion 24, 1989 Guidelines) by specifying clinical placements in sites where older adults are found under the supervision of faculty with gerontological expertise. The focus group asked for the assistance of the NLN representative present at this Gerontological Conference to present these concerns to the NLN Council of Baccalaureate and Higher Degree Programs. In addition, the group participants agreed to work collectively and individually to solicit support from the NLN.

2. *Experienced gerontological faculty in schools of nursing.* The support of deans and directors of schools of nursing is crucial in meeting this objective. The reality of budgetary cuts and the need to consider creative mechanisms was addressed. Geriatric Education Centers (GECs) are ideal sources to assist faculty members to attain or increase gerontological knowledge and identify appropriate student learning experiences. Joint appointments with gerontological clinical specialists or nurse practitioners is an additional source of expertise. Gerontological experts from clinical sites should be invited to join the curriculum committee to assist faculty with gerontological curriculum development.

3. *Specified theoretical and clinical content in each baccalaureate school of nursing.* The focus group felt no need to document specific content areas of gerontological nursing for this discussion. This content is clearly defined in the literature and textbooks. The group's aim was to share placement and quality of clinical learning experiences. There was no consensus as to placement of clinical experiences (sophomore, junior, or senior year) as students are successfully meeting objectives in each level of the nursing curriculum. The literature strongly reflects that student's

attitudes and ability to meet gerontological objectives is principally influenced by the faculty member's comfort and knowledge base in gerontological nursing. Faculty in attendance have been successful in multiple clinical sites. Students are involved with the well elderly in community sites and are providing care for the ill elderly in primary care settings, in the acute care setting and in long-term care settings, i.e., the nursing home, home health care or adult day care. Faculty feel that it is now essential to have specific learning experiences with the older adult in primary, secondary, and tertiary care settings because of the complexity of care required and the need to ascertain continuity of care for the older adult. Faculty believed that in order to maintain quality of the clinical experience, ongoing evaluation from both the nursing program and the clinical sites are necessary.

# 12

## Issues and Recommendations for Associate Degree Education in Gerontological Nursing

### Elaine Tagliareni

Conference participants representing Associate Degree Nursing education from New York to Hawaii met together to identify outcomes and strategies related to gerontological nursing integration. Initially, discussion centered on three timely and important questions.

*Where will we be teaching nursing?* Where are the best learning environments to understand both well and frail older adults? What nursing concepts related to older adults are best taught in each setting?

*What is the essential learning?* What body of knowledge is required to assist students to see older adults as unique individuals, to seek out rehabilitation potentials and to maintain and promote the older adult's optimal functional ability?

*How will we teach nursing?* What teaching strategies will facilitate care planning that is individualized and resident-focused? How can we best teach students to be caring professionals in a world "seized by technology" (Boyd, 1988).

As the discussion ensued, three major themes emerged. These themes became the foundation for identifying goals and determining strategies to advance gerontological nursing into the associate degree nursing curriculum.

1.  Acute care has become a transitional setting, not a landing place for cure.

2. It is vital for students to experience nursing care in a setting where they know clients "over time" in order to plan and evaluate care that is meaningful and individualized.

3. Current paradigms for clinical teaching may not be the most effective to assist students to individualize care and to follow through on the special needs of the older adult client.

The group formulated the following three goals with accompanying strategies:

**Goal:** Associate Degree students will individualize care to older adults; students will develop goals and interventions that relate to the person, not to the medical diagnosis.

**Strategies:** 1. Provide students with opportunities to plan care over time, i.e., long-term care, community settings. As students know clients over weeks, they will have time to evaluate and try new interventions. This activity will provide opportunities for creativity and give students the experience of making a difference in the care of older adults.

2. Develop care planning models where collaboration and creativity are valued and where students are encouraged to move beyond standardized plans. Some ideas included having students work in teams; use pencil or different color pens to write the care plans and cross-out and/or erase weekly; use the Minimum Date Set resident assessment instrument as the foundation for the care plan so students see operationalization of care plans.

3. Be a role model for students, both as a nurse who has positive regard for older adults and as a practitioner who values goals that relate to optimal functional ability, goals not necessarily found in a textbook.

4. Provide selected experiences for students in home settings to assist them to focus on the im-

pact of the older adult's home environment, on maintenance of independence, and to broaden their perspective on discharge planning.

**Goal**:    Associate Degree students will value the promotion of optimal functional ability for the older adult; specifically, students will combine physical, functional, and cognitive assessment to plan care directed toward promotion/maintenance of optimal functional ability.

**Strategies**:    1. Utilize long-term care settings, specifically nursing homes for clinical practice where the focus of nursing care is on prevention, health promotion, maintenance of function, seeking rehabilitation potentials, and sometimes cure.

2. Develop learning opportunities in the home setting to facilitate student understanding of how older adults function independently at home and how the home environment provides security and continuity for the older adult. This awareness has relevance for discharge planning and must include maintenance of function as well as medications and community referrals. Many of the participants utilize the well-elder experience developed by project schools in the W. K. Kellogg funded Community College Nursing Home Partnership (Waters, 1991).

3. Assist students to orient their thinking and care planning to maintenance of function in older adults. Faculty must encourage care planning directed toward walking, eating, toileting, grooming—self-care activities that promote independence and quality of life. In long-term care, the internationalization of chronic care goals can be difficult for students because it requires a different perspective. But it is an essential perspective if students are to be competent, health-promoting caregivers to older adults.

4. Develop teaching strategies to facilitate the transfer of learning from the nursing home to

other more technologically sophisticated settings, so that students recognize and promote optimal functional ability in all clinical situations where older adults are the major recipients of health care.

**Goal:** Faculty in Associate Degree Nursing Programs will engage in faculty development activities related to gerontological integration.

**Strategies:** 1. Recognize that most faculty have a limited background in gerontological nursing and that promoting interest and involvement in gerontology is an essential activity for all faculty groups.

2. Attend local and national conferences dealing with gerontological issues.

3. Provide opportunities for faculty to evaluate curriculum emphasis in gerontology, design new teaching strategies, and explore new clinical settings, where knowing individuals over time is possible.

Participants in the Associate Degree focus group are committed to inclusion of gerontological concepts in the nursing curriculum. Group members recognize that provision of safe and competent care to older adults requires a strong knowledge base in rehabilitation, maintenance of functional ability, and promotion of self-care, and that today, these practice patterns are nursing's privilege and responsibility.

## REFERENCES

Boyd, C. O. (1988). Phenomenology: A Foundation for Nursing Curriculum. In *Curriculum Revolution: Mandate for Change*, pp. 65-87. New York: National League for Nursing Press.

Waters, V. (Ed.). (1991). *Teaching Gerontology*. New York: National League for Nursing Press.

# 13

## Issues and Recommendations for Staff Development and Continuing Education in Gerontological Nursing

### Wanda R. Murray

This focus group provided a forum for discussion about issues related to staff development and continuing education in gerontological nursing. The group participants held backgrounds in nursing that included management, education, and clinical practice. To identify goals for the future of gerontological nursing as it relates to staff development and continuing education, key issues were identified that presently existed in gerontological nursing. These issues were 1) the professional image of the gerontological nurse, 2) clinical preparation of the gerontological nurse, and 3) management/administrative knowledge for the gerontological nurse.

Professional image of gerontological nurses was highlighted as an important area for continuing education and staff development. It is recognized that nurses employed in long-term care settings, in particular, have historically been perceived as having less skill, knowledge, and ambition than nurses practicing in other "more challenging" fields. It is also recognized that there is sometimes conflict between nursing home nurses and hospital nurses regarding their clinical expertise. The focus group members felt that this conflict was largely the result of a gap in knowledge and understanding of the roles and responsibilities that nurses assume in each of these practice settings. Efforts in staff development and continuing education need to address this misunderstanding. This can be achieved by promoting opportunities for greater dialogue and interchange among nurse and other health professionals involved in the care of the elderly in multiple practice settings. Such information sharing can contribute to a more positive image of the gerontological nurse.

Collaboration cannot be limited to just practice settings. It is also important to promote relationships between practice and education. Educators need to understand the skills and knowledge needed to provide care to older adults in a variety of practice settings so that future nurses can effectively function in these roles. Nursing faculty could collaborate with nurses in long-term care nursing facilities to develop continuing education programs for nursing faculty and nurse clinicians.

The focus group felt that it was essential to include the consumer in collaboration efforts. All health professionals must keep in touch with the needs of the clients they serve to continue to serve them well. Elder consumers could potentially lend a great deal of both popular and political support to the cause of gerontological nursing.

The members of the focus group were quite concerned that the emphasis on staff development and continuing education not be limited to registered nurses. Licensed practical nurses and nursing assistants play a vital role in providing care to older adults, particularly in long-term care facilities. Providing for their professional growth can only enhance the quality of care.

The second emphasis area was clinical preparation for the gerontological nurse. Many nurses currently employed in long-term care settings have not been educationally prepared to meet the challenges of that setting. One of the greatest deficits noted is physical assessment of the elder client. Nurses need assistance in learning how to perform mental status assessments and functional assessments. These skills are particularly important for nurses in long-term care settings to meet the intent of the newly implemented regulations from the Nursing Home Reform Act which requires that residents function at their highest practicable level possible.

Finally, the third emphasis area related to the education needs of nurse managers/administrators in settings for older adults. The group participants believed that nurse managers required more extensive knowledge in budgeting, strategic planning, cost-benefit analysis, product/service evaluation, and resource allocation. Continuing education offerings and staff development programs targeted to long-term care nurse administrators/managers are greatly needed.

# Part III

Abstracts of Poster and Roundtable Sessions

# A-1

## Adapting to Environmental Change:
## A Collaborative Practice Model

### Patricia A. Calico

One constant in today's practice environment is change. A recent change in long-term care settings was implementation of the OBRA (Omnibus Budget Reconciliation Act) requirement for nurse aide education. The Nurse Aide Training Program (NATP) requires 75 hours of initial nurse aide training and six hours of continuing education each quarter. The requirement was a challenge for many long-term care providers.

One facility conceptualized the change as an opportunity to expand the collaborative practice model. Introducing the collaborative model was a creative way of adapting to changes imposed upon the care setting by an outside agency. The change agent absorbed and diffused the tension created by change and the administration was distanced from the conflict of change while their NATP goals were achieved.

The facility and the university contractually arranged for the nurse educator joint appointment role to meet a facility need. The university was rewarded as well by enhancement of the gerontological nursing program. The success of the collaborative practice model sets a precedent for future joint projects.

# A–2

## Health Enhancement Nursing Clinical

### Barbara K. Andersen

Since the summer of 1984, faculty and students of The University of Tennessee at Chattanooga, School of Nursing have provided primary prevention nursing services in collaboration with Senior Neighbors of Chattanooga. Senior Neighbors of Chattanooga is organized to provide a variety of activities for the elderly to enhance their overall well-being and is also the coordinating agency for Title III-C nutrition programs. Approximately 2600 elderly are serviced through these combined programs. Community health faculty and the directors of several locations have met to identify self care needs of the elderly and ways that students can assist them to meet these needs. The goal has been to combine the community health clinical experience for senior citizens of the city of Chattanooga. In addition, it is expected that students will become more receptive to gerontological nursing concepts as a result of their experiences with the well elderly.

Nursing students and faculty provide a year-round nursing clinic at the Boynton Senior Neighbors Center which is located in the middle of seven low income high-rise apartment buildings for the elderly. Each week 40-to-50 clients attend the clinic for individual appointments with student nurses. They come to have their current health status monitored, to learn more about healthy lifestyles and/ or the care of identified health problems, and to talk with someone who provides an empathetic ear. The faculty member is available as an organizer, facilitator, and consultant. She also serves as a role model for assessing, teaching, and caregiving while providing needed foot care to other clients. In addition to weekly programs at the Boynton Center, foot care and screening programs for blood pressure, blood sugar, and cholesterol are also provided by students and faculty on a regular schedule to seven additional sites. Students collaborate with members of Senior Neighbors to identify common health concerns in order to present formal health related classes in various sites.

# A–3

## MDS+ Hotline Resource Person—A Service to Others

**Lois Obert**
**Mary Ann Santucci**
**Janet Feldman**

There is a unique learning experience in gerontological nursing presently taking place at Aurora University in Aurora, Illinois. This is due in part to one of the reforms called for by the Omnibus Budget Reconciliation Act of 1987 (OBRA) which mandates a uniform system to assess nursing home resident's ability to carry out daily life functions and identify significant impairments. One part of this assessment is the Minimum Data Set (MDS). An expanded approved version of the MDS, known as the MDS+, is now used in a Health Care Financing Administration (HCFA) funded research and demonstration project to test a resident information system and a resident classification system for equitable payment and for quality monitoring of process and outcomes adjusted for case mix. This project is the Multistate Nursing Home Case Mix and Quality Demonstration (NHCMQ) project. As part of the project, a hotline was established using Aurora University nursing students interested in gerontology, to help in gathering the data for classifying the nursing home residents. The five states using the MDS+ hotline are New York, Maine, Mississippi, South Dakota, and Kansas.

Initially, the purpose of the hotline was to provide a service, but it has resulted in being an invaluable educational experience for students. The interaction between the hotline worker and the caller leads to an exchange of ideas and problem solving which ultimately leads to the determination of a quality approach to the care of an individual resident. Stronger assessment skills develop during the interaction between health workers. The uniqueness of the learning comes from the interaction with the nurses and other health care workers in the facilities.

The MDS+ hotline is helping facilities to develop more consistent assessments. Sometimes callers have highly individualized interpretations of the various assessment items and need to understand how to think through the assessment task to answer the item in a compatible fashion. Maintaining a flexible attitude, understanding regional differences in nursing and long-term care practices and variations in state regulations, providing consistent definitions for the questions asked, and being an understanding listener for those frustrated by the assessment tasks is the hotline resource person's responsibility. Being able to carry out this task in a professional manner is an additional learning experience for these committed nursing students.

The MDS+ hotline is an exceptional learning experience for any nursing student. In essence, the student is helping shape the future of gerontological nursing by augmenting quality patient care.

# A–4

## The Community College–Nursing Home Partnership
## "Improving Care Through Education"

**Elaine Tagliareni**
**Ann Carignan**
**Mary Austin**

With funding from the W. K. Kellogg Foundation, a project called "The Community College–Nursing Home Partnership: Improving Care Through Education" has, since 1986, sponsored a variety of activities at six demonstration sites, in six states, to form partnerships between community college nursing programs and nursing homes. Nursing students in demonstration programs are taking redesigned and/or newly developed courses which focus on the healthy elderly as well as on the needs of the elderly in nursing home settings. Through selected research activities, faculty have determined "essential competencies" which are best taught in the nursing home, competencies which transfer to care of frail elders in all nursing care settings. Additionally, alliances between nursing home staff and faculty to improve quality of care have emerged at the demonstration sites.

# A–5

## Geropsychiatric Clinical Experiences in Long-Term Care

### Marianne Matzo

The Department of Nursing at Saint Anselm College in Manchester, New Hampshire, revised its curriculum and incorporated "gerontological strands" of content as part of a Health and Human Services, Division of Nursing Special Projects Grant (D10NU21084). These strands started in the first sophomore course and were built upon throughout the next three years. Students were receiving didactic information related to nursing considerations of the older adult without senior level experiential assignments.

In an effort to provide senior-level baccalaureate nursing students with the opportunity to have an innovative clinical experience in long-term care, a collaborative relationship was formed with the local county nursing home. The 400 bed facility was familiar with nursing students learning basic skills on its units, but never had advanced students for clinical experiences. The Director of Nursing was very interested in developing an advanced role for the nursing students and offered the home facilities for our use.

The long-term care (LTC) facility personnel worked very hard to prepare students' clinical experience. The students' clinical objectives were to facilitate a therapy and an activity group and to complete a comprehensive assessment of a confused elder. The students facilitated a "movement to music" activity program. To ensure continuity while the students were on semester breaks and over the summer, the Director of Nursing assigned activity personnel to the group. This staff member learned how to facilitate this group from the students and the clinical faculty person. The group now runs twice a week for the entire year.

Additionally, students facilitate a therapy group and choose their own modality (e.g., therapeutic reminiscing, art therapy, pet therapy). Activity staff were also assigned to this group so that they could learn about the different modalities. The activity staff are much more aware of a variety of therapeutic modalities than they had ever been before.

Evaluations of the experience were completed by the students at the end of each semester. The overwhelming positive responses to this experience have given it a firm place in the curriculum. The nursing staff appreciated the complete assessments and care plans that the students contribute. The Activity Department has become more creative and age-appropriate in their therapeutic programs. The students themselves are left with a positive impression of LTC and the therapeutic potential that this environment offers.

# A-6

## Collaboration between a Community College and a Social Service Agency: A Community-Based Practicum for Illness Prevention Among the Frail Elderly

Elizabeth Carey
Carolyn Cooper
Claire Wilcox

The Parkland College Nursing Department in Champaign, Illinois, developed a community clinical experience for Associate Degree nursing students that focused on illness prevention and health maintenance of elderly clients through a collaborative arrangement with Family Services of Champaign County, a Social Service Agency. Under a contractual arrangement, agency staff and faculty paired 83 students with frail elderly clients who were interested in a ten-week, one-hour home visiting program.

The main objectives of the experience were to increase student knowledge of functional health behaviors that enable the frail elderly to live at home; use nursing actions and communication skills that focused on illness prevention and health maintenance; increase understanding of a positive and mutually rewarding relationship between the nurse and elderly client; and to provide students an opportunity to collaborate with interdisciplinary team members and make referrals to community resources.

An analysis of the clinical objectives was based on student perceptions from weekly written logs (N = 830); a pre- and post-test of students' attitudes toward the elderly using the Kogan Attitudes Toward Old People Scale; nursing faculty supervision; and a midpoint final client evaluation with social workers.

Findings indicated student agreement that the health behaviors of mobility, recreation, using support systems, maintaining a positive self concept, and a stable physical status aided clients to live at home. Students collaborated with the social workers to link the client to social services for transportation or meals-on-wheels, and consulted with nursing faculty to link to Public Health or medical services. Eighty percent of the students reported understanding the professional work necessary to terminate with an elderly client dependent on community services; however, the Kogan questionnaire indicated no significant change in attitude toward the elderly. Fifty percent reported this experience offered more opportunity to provide health teaching than hospital clinical experiences.

# A–7

## Gerontic Nursing Education in a Community Hospital

Dianne Myers
Deborah Lautenslager

An institution-based continuing education/staff development model for gerontological nursing education entitled, *Gerontologic Nursing: Complexities of Caring for the Hospitalized Elderly* was developed two years ago and is taught monthly by the Gerontology Clinical Nurse Specialist of the Chambersburg Hospital in Chambersburg, Pennsylvania, for the nursing staff of a 217-bed rural community hospital. The primary goals of the course are (a) to affect attitudes toward empathetic understanding and advocacy for the elderly and (b) to enhance assessment skills toward more astute differentiations between manifestations of aging versus disease. Course content includes (a) aging simulation activities, (b) demographics and population trends, (c) theories of aging, (d) multiplicity, (e) ageism, (f) differentiation between normal age-related physiological changes and those changes resulting from common problems and pathology, (g) comparison between signs and symptoms of reversible and irreversible causes of confusion, (h) drugs and the elderly, (i) death and dying, and (j) ethical decision-making.

The end of course evaluation follows the standard requirements for any PNA (Pennsylvania Nurses Association) approved course. The six-month post-course evaluation is a qualitative questionnaire designed to determine if the course made a difference in attitudes toward and care of the elderly. Evaluations have been consistently positive with the most valuable parts of the course being information on age-related changes and confusion.

# A–8

## Nursing Student Experience: Aging in Place

Phyllis Armistead
Jessie Bryant

In July, 1989, Norfolk Redevelopment Housing Authority (NRHA) entered into an innovative collaborative agreement with Old Dominion University (ODU), School of Nursing to teach graduate and undergraduate nursing students about the health care needs of community-based older adults. This endeavor was funded, in part, by a Health and Human Services, Division of Nursing, Special Projects grant. Through this grant, NRHA employs a Gerontological Nurse Practitioner (GNP) that provides health care services to older adults in four mid-rise apartment complexes. The GNP coordinates student clinical experiences and serves as a clinical preceptor to students during the academic year.

Students have had a variety of experiences in the mid-rise apartments. Sophomore level students have done health assessments, physical examinations, and group wellness programs for the residents. Registered nurse students have used the clinical setting to learn about how individuals live and cope with chronic illnesses. Nurse practitioner students have their first experience in case management when they work with the GNP as a clinical preceptor. Nursing management of health programs and prevention of health problems can be emphasized in the nurse-managed setting.

Overall, students' response has been very positive. Knowledge of older persons' living arrangements, family situations, economic situations, and ability to function independently is used by the students when they care for older adults in acute care situations. The students' exposure to a role model with expertise in gerontological nursing has had many far-reaching benefits.

Perhaps the most exciting outcome, thus far, is the significant impact this partnership is making on the health care of older adults. Prior to 1989, NRHA provided no health related services. In one year, the services provided by the students and the GNP have contributed to improving the health status of many of the older residents in the mid-rises. In addition, other health and social services provided in the community are being utilized by the residents through the coordinating efforts on the part of the GNP and the students.

In summary, this collaborative arrangement between a community agency and a school of nursing has been beneficial to both parties. It provides students with clinical experience in a setting where there is a gerontological nurse role model and where nursing is truly practiced. It provides the residents with access to nursing and health care resulting in improved quality of life, while they "age in place."

# A–9

## Nursing Research in Long-Term Care: The Coler Memorial Hospital Model

Sarah Beaton
Annie Samuel
Carol Soto
Sharon Williams

The nursing research program at Coler Memorial Hospital on Roosevelt Island, in New York, was developed through a partnership of nurses from service and education facilitated by a staff member of the New York State Nurses Association. These nurses believed that the success of future gerontological nursing education, in both academic and practice setting rests with an increasing emphasis on nursing research. The conceptual framework for the model is derived from the legal definition of nursing elaborated in the ANA Social Policy Statement, Henderson's definition of nursing, the contrast between professional practice and QA (Quality Assurance) and agency-generated QA (Fielding and Beaton, 1992) and the work of Ida Orlando (1961/1990) whose question: "What happens to the patient as a result of the nurse's care?" guides many aspects of the program.

The first step for a nurse joining the nursing research team at Coler is to conduct a nursing diagnosis-intervention-resident outcome project. These projects, completed within a continuing education format, are seen as preludes to nursing research. The nurses are presented with the expectation that they can use their own knowledge, skill and creativity to improve the quality of care they deliver. They select a nursing diagnosis frequently occurring in their resident population, assess variables related to that diagnosis for a small group of residents, specify outcome objectives in measurable terms, plan and provide interventions, and systematically measure outcomes to evaluate efficacy of interventions.

To date, there have been three "waves" of projects, 21 projects completed by 28 nurses, some of whom worked in pairs. Twelve nurses dropped out before completing their work. Nurses who complete projects become mentors for nurses in subsequent waves, thus there is a spreading effect.

The projects also motivated interest in research. At the suggestion of the research team, composed of Coler nurses who complete projects and elect to stay involved, and faculty and graduate students from the education setting, a fourteen week course in nursing research was also offered at the facility. Nurses who completed the course received continuing education credits. Two graduate students, who had conducted nursing diagnosis-intervention-resident outcome projects during their graduate studies shared teaching responsibilities in this offering.

The current phase of the program includes plans for holding regularly scheduled nursing research critique forums and carrying out three rigorous studies with larger samples which build on earlier projects. In addition to the results of the projects—improved nursing practice and quality of life for residents evidenced by measurements of resident outcomes—other advantages of the collaboration include research-oriented staff development, enrichment and increased clinical relevance for the faculty member, and teaching and research experience for graduate students. Participating nurses reported "professional growth," "increased feelings of professional esteem," "new bonds among coworkers," and "increased pride in the facility." The need for large commitments of time within already crowded clinical and academic schedules is one major disadvantage identified.

## REFERENCES

Fielding, J., & Beaton, S. (1992). Quality assurance generated by professional nursing practice in long-term care. *Journal of Nursing Quality Assurance.* 6(2), 41–45.

Orlando, I. J. (1961/1990). *The dynamic nurse-patient relationship.* New York: National League for Nursing Press.

## A–10

### The Community College–Nursing Home Partnership

Mary Ann Anderson
Gerry Hansen

Weber State University (WSU) in Ogden, Utah, is a statewide nursing program that has educational programs for licensed practical nurses, associate degree registered nurses, and registered nurses seeking a baccalaureate degree. The school has six permanent campuses and three floating campuses that travel to rural areas of the state. At any one time, the nursing program has 550 student nurses in various levels of the educational process placed throughout the rural state of Utah.

With the demands of the national geriatric imperative and the nursing education call for a curriculum revolution that focuses on clinical experiences, WSU developed educational partnerships with 12 nursing facilities throughout the state. The purpose of these partnerships is to provide sound clinical learning experiences focused on the gerontological client at all student levels while providing quality care to the residents.

Each nursing home was selected because of its proximity to a WSU nursing program campus. It also is evaluated for administrative willingness to work with all levels of nursing students and faculty, the ability to pass state survey well, and the presence of registered nurse role-models. Once the nursing program administration makes the initial contact with the nursing facility and negotiates the legal concerns regarding contracts and liability, a nursing faculty member is assigned to the facility as a liaison person.

The liaison person is responsible for establishing and maintaining a positive relationship with the nursing home administration staff. This is a serious commitment on the part of the faculty person. Other faculty members realize that any communication, concerns, or questions regarding a partnership home are to be directed to the liaison faculty member.

After four years, 11 of the original 12 partnership homes are still functioning. Nursing home staff are regularly assigned to teach in management classes and on issues panels. The nursing students report positive learning experiences and faculty are beginning to function comfortably in the new setting. Some students are asking to have preceptorships in the LTC (Long-Term Care) facilities. All of these behaviors are seen as methods for meeting the demands of both the geriatric imperative and the call for a curriculum revolution.

# A–11

## *Education and Practice: An Eclectic Model*

**Sandie Engberg**
**Barbara Smith**
**Barbara Spier**
**Ann Yurick**
**Martha Meis**
**Linda Organist**

At the University of Pittsburgh, School of Nursing, multiple models of collaboration have been developed for teaching gerontological nursing at the graduate and undergraduate levels. These models have been influenced by the philosophy of the School of Nursing, which values the promotion, restoration, and maintenance of health throughout the life span; undergraduate and graduate curriculum designs; and clinical settings representative of cultural and ethnic diversity of the elderly population in the urban and surrounding areas. The undergraduate program includes health promotion with clinical experience in health assessment and health education in elderly apartment buildings and senior centers. Of much importance is the collaborative relationship of the managers of these settings with the faculty. Following the clinical experience with the well elderly, the undergraduate student cares for the frail elderly in an institutionalized setting. One model includes faculty collaboration with a gerontological nursing clinical specialist who serves as a resource person; promotes interdisciplinary team planning; and serves as a link between faculty and other clinical services in a nursing home setting. In another model, a faculty member provides students with learning experiences in a nursing home and on a geriatric unit of an acute care setting during the term. This faculty is a member of the Board of Directors in the nursing home. Student experience with elderly in a nursing home and in acute care provides comparison of care in different types of settings and an opportunity to participate in planning for continuity of care as an elderly person returns to the community.

The graduate program prepares the geriatric nurse practitioner. Clinical experience is provided at the Benedum Geriatric Assessment Center of the University Health Center. Geriatric nurse practitioners employed in this setting serve as preceptors for their graduate students. The faculty member responsible for this course uses this assessment center as a practice site and is familiar with the clients, staff, and services. For students, opportunity is provided for health assessment and health promotion in the assessment center; participation in a Continence Program; practice in a setting with interdisciplinary services and research opportunities; and opportunity for home visits. Student research requirement can be part of ongoing research at this assessment center.

# A–12

## Determining Future Educational Trends
## for Undergraduate Nursing Education
## in Ontario, Canada

**Anne Beckingham**
**Olga Roman**
**Gaye Graves**
**Alfreda Kartha**

This presentation describes the Educational Center for Aging and Health (ECAH) at McMaster University, Hamilton, Ontario. This provincial center for excellence in gerontology has as its overall mission, two major facets:

1. To increase the number and proportion of skilled health professionals who are committed to *promoting health* and providing excellent care for aging individuals; and

2. To develop collaborative, *interdisciplinary*, and interprofessional educational approaches and models concerning aging and health, and evaluating their effectiveness.

One of the five major components of ECAH is the Provincial Network, which encompasses the activities of the Ontario University Coalition for Education in Health Care of the Elderly, and annual conferences on "Education in Aging and Health for Ontario." These two initiatives bring together faculty members active in geriatric and gerontological education and research, as well as government and community leaders. Nursing educational issues of concern province-wide have been addressed in order to enhance communication, to share McMaster's progress in innovative inter-professional education, to facilitate collaboration and partnership between university programs, and to monitor progress through education, toward the achievement of the long-term goals of promoting healthy aging.

The Coalition for Education in Health Care of the Elderly initiates a series of discipline-specific working groups to review gerontological content in health sciences education. Representatives from nine Ontario degree granting school of nursing programs have met to plan for and develop gerontological nursing guidelines for curriculum change. This discipline-specific group has met on several occasions, guided by the mandate:

*"To develop a province-wide-network to plan for the educational content in undergraduate degree programs in the promotion of Aging and Health."*

The group did a critical analysis of documented curricula, reviewed (inter)national literature on education and the future role of the gerontological nurse, and the process of curriculum construction. Through consensus decision-making, a Position Paper on gerontological nursing curriculum with strategies for implementation is being finalized.

# A–13

## A Small Wellness Clinic for Colorado Seniors: An Excellent Collaborative Experience for the University of Colorado

**Alice F. Running**
**Anne Harrison**

In the late 1970s or early 1980s members of the community of Brighton, Colorado contacted the School of Nursing at the University of Colorado Health Sciences Center (UCHSC) to request nursing services for the seniors of Brighton. A formal contract was written between the UCHSC–School of Nursing and the city of Brighton, allowing the School of Nursing to charge for the services they provided. Brighton Senior Center and the city of Brighton pay an annual fee to the UCHSC–School of Nursing. Since the opening of the clinic, a nurse practitioner has staffed a weekly wellness clinic. Services provided to the seniors by the nurse practitioner include physical examinations, blood pressure checks, blood glucose checks, pedicures, health education, and health promotion. Statistics showing utilization of the clinic by seniors are now available for the years 1988–1990 and they are as follows: 1) in 1988 a total of 1,522 visits were made to the clinic, 2) in 1989 a total of 1,163 visits were made, and 3) in 1990 a total of 1,250 visits were made to the clinic.

Approximately 10–12 students from the UCHSC–School of Nursing Primary Care of Adults Masters program are able to obtain clinical experience from the clinic each year, enabling them to improve their geriatric assessment and interpersonal relationship skills.

The School of Nursing at UCHSC is grounded on a philosophy of caring, and a philosophy such as this requires that the practitioner, student, and senior enter into a relationship that is based on client advocacy. The Brighton clinic allows the practitioner and student to truly interact with the senior seeking health care. A relationship is developed that can foster health promotion. This health promotion must include the senior's perception of description of health. The weekly clinic is able to provide continuity of care to the seniors, and is an excellent setting for practitioners and students to realize how rewarding it is to provide health care for this population.

# A–14

## Bridging the Gap
## between Education and Practice:
## Experiences Teaching Gerontological Nursing

### Virginia Brooke

The Intercollegiate Center for Nursing Education, in Spokane, Washington, offers a three semester credit elective course in Gerontological Nursing. It is offered to baccalaureate and graduate students, and staff nurses from nursing homes, hospitals, and home health agencies. The challenge is to meet the needs of students at various levels of educational preparation from various areas of practice while maintaining a standard of academic rigor. Course objectives and learning experiences bridge education and practice by developing the student nurse beside the staff nurse.

Course objectives direct students to: 1) evaluate the nurse's role in a variety of settings; 2) analyze selected physical, emotional, and social problems of the elderly; 3) study effective nursing interventions; and 4) discuss major legislation and social programs for the elderly. An additional objective for graduate students is to: 5) evaluate current published research on nursing care of the elderly. Students in 483 and 583 share one hour of lecture and 3 hours of clinical assignment weekly. One hour of seminar is offered separately to each group of students.

Clinical assignments designed around the course objectives and promoting integration of practice and theory are completed by students in their respective agencies. An example of clinical assignment on the sub-objective on medications is: "Estimate the anticholinergic exposure from the drug regime of two patients in our agency using the formula in Chenitz, 1991, p. 385." Seminar discussion follows the experience. An assigned paper, which includes an annotated bibliography, describes a current or projected project to deal with a problem identified in the student's agency. Graduate students are expected to integrate more research in the paper.

The following advantages resulting from the course are: 1) greater depth in theory and practice; 2) networking experiences between staff and student nurses; 3) interaction between staff and faculty member resulting in consultation between educator and practitioner; 4) encouragement of student nurses and staff nurses to continue working toward a baccalaureate or master's degree; and 5) identification of problematic areas of practice.

# A–15

## Gerontology and Introduction to Nursing Management

### Mary Ann Kolis

The last course in the Associate Degree Nursing Program in Gateway Technical College in Kenosha, Wisconsin, is Gerontology and Introduction to Nursing Management. This four-credit course provides opportunities for students to integrate gerontology theories into meeting basic needs and altered health states of older adults. Management principles and strategies are introduced at a beginning level. Learning takes place through a competency based curriculum with implementation of varied learning strategies in the classroom, auto-tutorial laboratory, and clinical practicum.

The theory content is presented in the first two weeks—four days per week. In the past two semesters, six nursing homes—three in Kenosha, two in Racine, and one in Elkhorn were used as clinical facilities for approximately fifty students. The students are in clinical three days per week, eight hours each day, for four weeks. During the first eight-hour day of clinical, the students work with the nursing assistants and complete one Geriatric Nursing History/Assessment in order to acclimate themselves to the setting. For the remainder of the clinical time, each student begins team leading with four clients the first week and then advances to approximately ten to twelve clients by their last clinical week. The students also observe resident care conferences, rehabilitation services, and the different roles of nursing staff and administration within the nursing home setting. As an observational experience, the students visit an adult day care center and a senior center to acquaint themselves with the available community resources for the elderly.

# A–16

## Gerontology as a Focus
## for Traditional and Non-Traditional
## Approaches to Nursing Education

Joan M. Culley
Janet A. Courtney

Holyoke Community College (HCC), in Holyoke, Massachusetts, has in place two career options for students pursuing an Associate Degree in Nursing, that provide a curriculum that meets the needs of a diverse student population and provide clinical experience that focuses on the health care needs of the elderly. HCC has both a traditional day school program and an alternative non-traditional career pathway (*Nursing Career Pathway Program*) in collaboration with Regents College in Albany, New York. The faculty were aware of the acute need to educate nurses in the care of the elderly and opted to employ a full-time faculty member who specializes in this area of care and teaching. Over eight years ago, HCC developed a five week gerontology clinical experience in a local nursing home. All traditional nursing students rotate through this experience during their second or third semester. Through the expertise developed and the interest in meeting the needs of the growing elderly population, HCC implemented strategies in both career options that incorporate gerontology nursing into the curriculum.

The majority of students recruited into the Nursing Career Pathway Program are employees of long-term care facilities. Approximately fifty percent of the students enrolled are employees of Genesis Health Ventures (a chain of long-term care facilities in the Northeast). Genesis Health Ventures fully supports, funds, and mentors these selected employees through the Nursing Career Pathway Program. HCC, Regents College, and Genesis Health Ventures work together to provide support services and opportunities that will enable these employees to be successful and remain in long-term care as Registered Nurses. It is possible to utilize learning opportunities with the elderly in these long-term care institutions, to provide the link between theory and practice. In this way, students learn more about gerontological nursing and the application of basic nursing skills to the specific needs of the elderly. A key component of the program is that it is a gerontological nursing experience which provides a wide variety of learning opportunities where most nursing skills and knowledge can be both learned and applied.

Along with several Western Massachusetts Community Colleges, HCC was selected as a cluster member school for a W. K. Kellogg Foundation Grant. This grant provides on-going support to program faculty as they engage in curriculum study to include active preparation of graduates for nursing roles in gerontology and long-term care. Member colleges examine data regarding what students can best learn in long-term nursing home settings, review variables that contribute to the success of a partnership, and engage in discussion regarding the validity of curriculum redirection. This project began in the Fall of 1991.

# A–17

## Faculty Practice in Long-Term Care Setting: A Collaborative Model

Brenda L. Cleary
Dorothy Jackson

Teaching nursing homes have been hailed as a success story nationwide. Even in less populated areas with more limited resources, many of the concepts of the teaching nursing home can be implemented. A collaborative arrangement between Seabury Center Nursing Care Unit and Texas Tech University Health Sciences Center (TTUHSC) School of Nursing in the Permian Basin, both of which are located in Odessa, Texas, was developed to implement the teaching nursing home concepts.

A faculty practice evolved early in 1991 when a board member of Seabury Center Nursing Care Unit, a 97-bed not-for-profit institution operated by St. John's Episcopal Church in Odessa, Texas, recognized the need for additional gerontological clinical expertise in the faculty. The board member, who is a nurse educator and Chairperson of Nursing at Odessa College, also had future aims of involving associate nursing students in the facility and wanted some guidance and direction in that area. Seabury contracted TTUHSC School of Nursing in the Permian Basin for the services of the Associate Dean who is a clinical nurse specialist (CNS).

At the present time, the CNS provides four hours per week in the nursing home facility which involves patient assessment and nursing care planning, quality assurance and implementation of minimum data sets, risk management including wound care and prevention and fall prevention, and specific consultation regarding dementia care, as well as management and communication issues.

The functional aspects of the CNS include direct patient care and assessment, attending and guiding multi-disciplinary care planning sessions, role modeling, and providing inservice education. This collaborative arrangement has also evolved to represent a partnership between education and practice with the involvement of both ADN students and RN-BSN students.

Multi-disciplinary care planning sessions have changed directions in a very meaningful way. Walking rounds are now conducted prior to the initiation of the care planning session. Both residents and family members are more involved in the process. A nursing assistant is being added as a participant in the sessions and the conduct of the meetings involves a greater use of minimum data sets in initiating the discussion of care needs. Chart audits are conducted by the director of nursing and the CNS.

Other outcomes measures include staff and board satisfaction, positive inservice evaluations, and positive student evaluations of the nursing home as a clinical agency. It is evident that there is better management of residents with dementia which typically represent a large percentage of the resident population in nursing homes. Long-range goals include improved risk management and improvement in state surveys.

# A–18

## Continuing Education for Nurses in Geriatric Home Care

Shannon Patton
Marilyn Pattillo

A shift in the delivery of care to elders from the hospital to the community has resulted in an increased client acuity in the home care setting. Both experienced and new community health nurses are challenged to provide acute care skills and make independent decisions in a different context. To meet these challenges, a continuing education series of seven workshops, funded by the Department of Health and Human Services, is being offered at three sites in Texas. Its purpose is threefold: 1) to upgrade nurses' theoretical knowledge and clinical skills in geriatrics; 2) to provide new home care nurses with theory in community health; and 3) to provide experienced home health nurses with up-to-date acute care skills.

A collaborative effort between the grant and community home care agencies has contributed to the success of this project. Initially, home care agencies were surveyed state-wide to inquire about their interest and need for continuing education in geriatric home care. All respondents (72 percent response rate) confirmed the need and supported the project. Agencies asked that workshop content be practical in nature, accessible, and at a low cost. As a result, workshop content was designed for the practicing nurse and includes content on physiological changes of aging, psychosocial issues and aging, chronicity, home care concepts, case management, and intravenous and respiratory care skills. In addition, five home-study modules have been produced which addressed nutrition, confusion, caring for caregivers, stroke and incontinence.

Four home care agencies in the Austin area participated in the first year of the project. Interviews of the nursing director and a nurse representative from each agency provided valuable input for the development of workshop content and a learning needs assessment tool. The evaluation component of the project has included written participant evaluations (perception of mastery), participant background information, interviews of pilot nurses and their supervisors, and follow-up surveys.

Working with the Center for Health Care Research and Evaluation at The University of Texas at Austin, School of Nursing, a learning needs assessment (pre- and post-test) was developed and tested the first grant year. The product is an 86-item pretest which will be used in the second grant year to identify knowledge deficits of pilot group nurse participants.

During the second grant year, each of the four pilot agencies will administer the pretest to at least five nurses. Based on the test results, nurses will be scheduled for the appropriate learning activity (workshop). Nurses unable to attend the assigned workshop have the option of viewing the workshop videotapes. All pilot nurse participants will complete a participant background questionnaire, self-evaluation of mastery of objectives, post-test, and a follow-up interview.

# A–19

## Maximizing Gerontological Resources in the Acute Care Setting

M. Catherine Wollman
Michael Clark
Mary Ann Haggerty

At the University of Pennsylvania, undergraduate junior nursing students take a seven week course entitled "Nursing Practice with the Older Adult." The primary clinical focus in this course is the acute care setting in order to prepare students to meet the increasingly complex changes that older adults present within the hospital system.

Faculty identified three levels of clinical involvement that would be necessary for ongoing stability and quality of course and clinical content:

1.  Highly qualified clinical faculty with gerontological experience;

2.  Resource personnel to complement the classroom and clinical experience;

3.  Selection of hospital units which would provide high intensity of older adults and opportunities for critical thinking.

Clinical faculty have included: primary care, geriatric nurse practitioners who were gerontological experts but not as familiar with the acute care setting; master's prepared hospital staff with joint positions with the school of nursing; and master's prepared hospital staff who functioned as "master teachers" assuming the role of clinical teachers for one or two students while continuing in their usual role. Frequent clinical faculty meetings and clinical site visits from gerontological faculty have allowed the hospital based clinical instructors to integrate classroom content and specified gerontological objectives at a consistently high level.

Resource personnel continue to be identified in order to achieve high level of synthesis of course content which includes: Health system issues affecting the older adult; Comprehensive assessment; Common medical surgical problems affecting older people; and principals of continuity of care and discharge planning, rehabilitation, pharmacodynamics, ethics and clinical research.

Resource personnel include nurse clinical specialists in orthopedics, cancer, incontinence, rehabilitation, cardiovascular, and respiratory content. Physical and occupational therapists have contributed strongly to the knowledge base of functional status. Discharge planners and discharge planning rounds stress the need for discharge planning from the first day of hospitalization. Pharmacists have been asked to present the special problems of older adults due to polypharmacy, costs, and commonly prescribed drugs. Nurse researchers who have used the hospital setting to study restraint issues, delirium and discharge planning have also presented their findings.

Certain hospital units lend themselves to integration of specific content. The orthopedic floor provides rich experiences in exploring falls, functional status, rehabilitation, discharge planning, and use of the interdisciplinary team. The medical units necessitate consideration of polypharmacy, sensory deficits, multiple chronic problems of frail elderly and placement issues. The surgical units present older adults with delirium, use of restraints, and multiple ethical issues.

The introduction of a specific gerontological course and acute care clinical experience has heightened the awareness of students and hospital personnel to the challenges offered by the older adult in this setting.

# A–20

## *Center for ElderHealth*

**Linda E. Moody**
**Katherine Echevarria**
**Joan Bezon**

The Center for ElderHealth is a nurse-directed clinic sponsored by the Department of Gerontology Nursing at the University of South Florida. It operates in collaborative arrangement with the Tampa House Authority for low-income elderly who live in a medically underserved area in Tampa, Florida. The state health department was involved in providing educational materials and partial funding for the project. The majority of the elderly who are served by this free standing clinic are Hispanic. The majority of elderly seen in the clinic has no form of private or federal health insurance coverage. The purpose of the Center is to provide quality health care services for the underserved and a quality learning environment for gerontology nurse practitioner graduate students, their practice, and directed research.

The collaboration permits the gerontology nursing faculty to better socialize gerontology graduate nursing students to their advanced practice role in an innovative setting, whereby they can implement and validate their practitioner skills, and at the same time provide a valuable and needed service to an underserved group of elderly. It also provides a rich setting for students and faculty to conduct research.

Students gain experience in health assessment by using the ElderHealth Profile (Moody, 1990). It is a comprehensive question-naire which assesses health risk measures in persons over age 55, including health history, health utilization and health status, functional status, depression, mastery, and quality of life. Basic demographic data are also obtained. Other health assessment data are collected (blood pressure, height, weight, and medication history) which are entered into the computer data base. The first version of the software program was developed, tested, and evaluated for English speaking elders, then converted with the means of a Spanish translation program for use with Hispanic elderly groups.

# A-21

## Innovations in Gerontological Nursing Education: The Hospital Based Gerontological Nurse Specialist as Consultant to Baccalaureate Nursing Students

**Lori Hasty**
**Fay Sims**

Traditionally baccalaureate nursing students have a number of client care assignments with older individuals in the acute care setting. However, the focus of the clinical experience has not been gerontological nursing.

This project developed by Old Dominion University, School of Nursing and funded by the U.S. Department of Health and Human Services, Division of Nursing is based on the collaboration between the School of Nursing and the acute care hospital, as a model site for student affiliations. The gerontological nurse specialist employed by Chesapeake General Hospital served as a "consultant clinical instructor" to students and the students' clinical instructor from the university. A number of strategies were employed to meet the learning needs of the students. Outcomes of this experience have been favorable. Students and staff have gained valuable knowledge in caring for the older client. Staff examples include a significant increase in documentation of the plan of care regarding skin integrity and increased GNS consultation. Student examples include increased understanding of the role of the professional nurse in caring for older hospitalized clients, increased consideration of gerontological nursing as a specialty after graduation, and increased recognition of the health related needs of the older hospitalized client.

# A–22

## *Life Span: Interdisciplinary Partnerships–*
## *The Nursing Perspective*

**Kay T. Roberts**
**Beverly E. Holland**
**Keith R. Knapp**
**Kathy D. Shireman**

Life Span is a unique, innovative approach to interdisciplinary collaboration. Based upon the concept of partnerships, the program brings educators, service providers, and persons from business sectors together to develop model health care delivery programs. The purpose of the Life Span Interdisciplinary Curriculum is to prepare undergraduate and graduate students from nursing, medicine, social work, physical therapy, and dentistry to implement successful interdisciplinary health care teams that will assess, plan, and evaluate care of older adults. The curriculum encompasses an interdisciplinary, faculty-supervised, four-week rotation with 20 hours of team collaboration regarding older adult clients from the nursing home, a congregate living site, and the community setting. The rotation begins with didactic and experiential activities related to team dynamics. Students conduct comprehensive assessment of older adults and plan and conduct team conferences for these clients. The students present the plan of care to the primary nurse to mutually validate or revise the plan. Students have practice in using technology to communicate with members of a "distant" team, e.g., FAX, electronic mail, and conducting telephone conferences.

# A–23

## Partnerships between Nursing Students and Nursing Home Staff Through Nursing Research

Sandra Karam
Marguerite White
Denise M. Nies

In response to the rapid growth in the frail elderly population and to the need for professional nurses who have a strong educational foundation in gerontology to care for this population, Beth Sholom Home of Eastern Virginia (BSHEV) and the Old Dominion University School of Nursing entered an exciting partnership to provide undergraduate nursing students with a creative and innovative clinical experience in a nursing home setting. This partnership was supported by funding from a three year Special Projects Grant from the Division of Nursing, U.S. Department of Health and Human Services. The Model Gerontological Clinical Sites (MGCS) project funded a Gerontological Nurse Specialist (GNS) that was employed by the home to provide advanced nursing services to the residents and to serve as a clinical preceptor for nursing students. The GNS and nursing faculty worked together to develop many unique learning experiences, one of which involved staff and students in solving a clinical problem through nursing research. After conducting a needs assessment with nursing home staff and administration, the GNS identified resident bowel incontinence, constipation, and dependent laxative usage as a long-standing problem. Based on research literature supporting bowel management programs, a clinical objective was developed to address the implementation of a program to decrease laxative dependency and improve natural bowel functioning. The design of a clinical teaching strategy that combined the steps of assessment, planning, intervention and evaluation with the primary steps of the research process, provided students and staff with a blueprint with which to create an empirically-based, realistic bowel management program.

The outcome of the bowel management program has resulted in positive changes at the nursing facility in bowel management protocols. All tube fed residents are now receiving formulas containing fiber. Assessments are conducted on all residents prior to admission in order to develop individualized bowel programs. The house bowel regime has been revised to reflect more natural bowel functioning resulting in reduced laxative usage.

# A–24

## Professionalism and Creativity in Gerontological Nursing Education

### Patricia A. Calico

Increasing numbers of older persons with diverse and complex health care needs require that nurses be educationally and experientially prepared to address the health care challenges in gerontological nursing. The University of Cincinnati College of Nursing and Health and Maple Knoll Village Robert Wood Johnson Teaching Nursing Home Project marked the beginning of collaboration to establish a Gerontological Nursing Care Model for education and practice at Maple Knoll Village. One decade later graduate and undergraduate student nurses are an integral part of the practice environment, Maple Knoll Village residents are primary teachers, and education is a norm throughout the retirement village. Two Gerontological Clinical Nurse Specialists with joint faculty/practitioner appointments are liaisons between practice and education.

Assumptions of the Gerontological Nursing Model are that aging is a normal developmental process and that individuals uniquely experience aging. Further, aging is conceptualized as an intricately woven tapestry intertwining threads of feelings, thoughts, desires and actions, which becomes richer as life threads are added. It is this essence of aging that students are guided to capture in the professional practice model.

Teaching/learning strategies consistent with the professional model include an initial clinical experience with well older adults in an independent living arrangement, with progression to caring for residents with dependent care needs. Interdisciplinary learning with health care professional students in medicine and pharmacy expand student problem solving skills. Affective learning is gauged by applying the arts. Students write a Haiku, a form of Japanese poetry to express feelings about aging and care of the older adult. Graduate students assist in research and initiate practice projects to improve quality care.

Many advantages are realized as a result of the collaboration between the College of Nursing and Maple Knoll Village. Education and practice setting missions are fulfilled in the provision of quality resident care. Faculty and staff develop an expertise in gerontological practice and education and foster student learning in a positive and nurturing environment. Older adults are active participants in the teaching/learning process and derive self-growth from their generativity. Interdisciplinary collaboration is practiced and students engage in critical thinking and problem solving. Research is conducted for the purposes of improving practice outcomes and knowledge and is disseminated through publications. Standards of care are high and creativity flourishes among all members of the healthcare team in the maintenance of quality resident care and the discovery of gerontological nursing as an exciting and rewarding practice area.

# A–25

## Gerontologic Nursing Education Continuing Care Program

Marjorie Maddox
Lorraine Guida

In 1975, the American Nurses Association began to advocate for the inclusion of gerontological nursing in the undergraduate curriculum. Recently, the need was emphasized again in the recommendations stated in the final report of the Commission on Nursing of the U.S. Department of Health and Human Services. Georgetown University, School of Nursing in Washington, DC, responded to this documented need by developing a four-year integrated continuing care approach to incorporating gerontological nursing into the undergraduate curriculum.

Realizing the planning of a four-year integrated approach would require the unique blend of the "right" clinical settings plus capable faculty prepared in gerontology, the project faculty was carefully chosen. A variety of clinical agencies was represented with each member being appointed to adjunct faculty status. Agency faculty members included representation from adult day care, visiting nurse agencies, nursing homes, a rehabilitation hospital, and the in-hospital geriatric medical specialty care unit at Georgetown University Hospital.

The challenge was to find the best methods of preparing nursing students to understand and address the needs of the elderly population. Nursing knowledge and skill must be employed to care not only for the acutely ill, but also to promote health and to promote health maintenance and rehabilitation. To do this, the educational experiences must include both acute and community care. That was a basic assumption. But, how could this best be done within the tightly scheduled baccalaureate curriculum, where the focus has often been primarily on acute hospital high-technology care, not necessarily with a strong focus on the aging person? The use of the continuum of care proved to be the answer, but the value of these types of clinical experiences must be convincingly demonstrated not only to the students but also to the faculty.

The gerontology project has provided the resources to integrate service and practice. The adjunct faculty from the agencies, who are an integral part of the project staff, supplement the real world dimensions of the faculty with an in-depth understanding of each of their agencies or facilities and patients/clients. The graduates of the nursing program are prepared to function with the older adult having a practical understanding of the fiscal issues that affect service provisions and a broad knowledge base regarding the services that constitute a continuum of care.

One outgrowth of this project was an Invitational National Competencies Consensus Conference held in Fall, 1990. Following the initial efforts, the members of the project faculty worked with the competency statements to develop AD, BSN, and MSN gerontological nursing competencies. The final product was published by the National League for Nursing as *Gerontology in the Nursing Curriculum*.